Salvage Therapies for Non-Muscle Invasive Bladder Cancer

Editor

BADRINATH R. KONETY

UROLOGIC CLINICS
OF NORTH AMERICA

www.urologic.theclinics.com

Consulting Editor
SAMIR S. TANEJA

February 2020 • Volume 47 • Number 1

ELSEVIER

1600 John F. Kennedy Boulevard • Suite 1800 • Philadelphia, Pennsylvania, 19103-2899

http://www.theclinics.com

UROLOGIC CLINICS OF NORTH AMERICA Volume 47, Number 1
February 2020 ISSN 0094-0143, ISBN-13: 978-0-323-72256-8

Editor: Kerry Holland
Developmental Editor: Laura Kavanaugh

Urologic Clinics of North America (ISSN 0094-0143) is published quarterly by Elsevier Inc., 360 Park Avenue South, New York, NY 10010-1710. Months of issue are February, May, August, and November. Business and Editorial Offices: 1600 John F. Kennedy Blvd., Suite 1800, Philadelphia, PA 19103-2899. Periodicals postage paid at New York, NY and additional mailing offices. Subscription prices are $391.00 per year (US individuals), $795.00 per year (US institutions), $100.00 per year (US students and residents), $450.00 per year (Canadian individuals), $993.00 per year (Canadian institutions), $100.00 per year (Canadian students/residents), $520.00 per year (foreign individuals), $993.00 per year (foreign institutions), and $240.00 per year (foreign students/residents). Foreign air speed delivery is included in all *Clinics* subscription prices. All prices are subject to change without notice. **POSTMASTER:** Send address changes to *Urologic Clinics of North America*, Elsevier Health Sciences Division, Subscription Customer Service, 3251 Riverport Lane, Maryland Heights, MO 63043. **Customer Service: 1-800-654-2452 (US). From outside the United States, call 1-314-447-8871. Fax: 1-314-447-8029. E-mail: JournalsCustomerServiceusa@elsevier.com (for print support)** and **JournalsOnlineSupport-usa@elsevier.com (for online support).**

Reprints. For copies of 100 or more, of articles in this publication, please contact the Commercial Reprints Department, Elsevier Inc., 360 Park Avenue South, New York, New York 10010-1710. Tel.: 212-633-3874; Fax: 212-633-3820; E-mail: reprints@elsevier.com.

Urologic Clinics of North America is covered in MEDLINE/PubMed (*Index Medicus*), *Excerpta Medica, Current Contents/Clinical Medicine, Science Citation Index,* and *ISI/BIOMED*.

Contributors

CONSULTING EDITOR

SAMIR S. TANEJA, MD
The James M. Neissa and Janet Riha Neissa
Professor of Urologic Oncology, Professor of
Urology, Radiology, and Biomedical
Engineering, GU Program Leader, Perlmutter
Cancer Center, Director, Division of Urologic
Oncology, Department of Urology, NYU
Langone Health, New York, New York, USA

EDITOR

BADRINATH R. KONETY, MD, MBA, FACS
Professor and Dougherty Family Chair in
Urologic Oncology, Department of Urology,
Vice Dean for Clinical Affairs, University of
Minnesota Medical School, Chief Executive
Officer, University of Minnesota Physicians,
Chief Clinical Officer, MHealth Fairview,
University of Minnesota, Minneapolis,
Minnesota, USA

AUTHORS

JOHANNES ALFRED WITJES, PhD
Department of Urology, Radboud University
Nijmegen Medical Centre, Nijmegen, The
Netherlands

TOM J.H. ARENDS, PhD
Department of Urology, Canisius-Wilhelmina
Ziekenhuis, Nijmegen, The Netherlands

RUSSELL E.N. BECKER, MD, PhD
Department of Urology, The Greenberg
Bladder Cancer Institute, Brady Urological
Institute, Johns Hopkins Hospital, Baltimore,
Maryland, USA

TRINITY J. BIVALACQUA, MD, PhD
Department of Urology, The Greenberg
Bladder Cancer Institute, Brady Urological
Institute, Johns Hopkins Hospital, Baltimore,
Maryland, USA

ALBERTO BREDA, MD
Department of Urology, Fundacion Puigvert,
Autonomous University of Barcelona,
Barcelona, Spain

NATHAN A. BROOKS, MD
Department of Urology, The University of Iowa
Hospitals and Clinics, Iowa City, Iowa,
USA

CARISSA E. CHU, MD
Department of Urology, University of California,
San Francisco, San Francisco, California,
USA

LAUREN FOLGOSA COOLEY, MD, PhD
Department of Urology, Northwestern
University, Feinberg School of Medicine,
Polsky Urologic Cancer Institute, Chicago,
Illinois, USA

COLIN P.N. DINNEY, MD
Department of Urology, The University of
Texas MD Anderson Cancer Center, Houston,
Texas, USA

ÓSCAR RODRÍGUEZ FABA, MD
Department of Urology, Fundacion Puigvert,
Autonomous University of Barcelona,
Barcelona, Spain

GARY D. GROSSFELD, MD, MPH
Bristol-Myers Squibb, Lawrenceville, New
Jersey, USA

SHILPA GUPTA, MD
Department of Hematology and Oncology,
Taussig Cancer Institute, Cleveland Clinic
Foundation, Cleveland, Ohio, USA

CHRISTOPHER R. HAAS, MD
Columbia University Department of Urology,
Herbert Irving Pavilion, New York, New York,
USA

JEFFREY HOLZBEIERLEIN, MD, FACS
Professor and Chair, Department of Urology,
The University of Kansas Medical Center,
Kansas City, Kansas, USA

BRANT A. INMAN, MD, MS
Division of Urology, Duke University Medical
Center, Durham, North Carolina, USA

ASHISH M. KAMAT, MD
Department of Urology, The University of
Texas MD Anderson Cancer Center, Houston,
Texas, USA

MAX R. KATES, MD
Department of Urology, The Greenberg
Bladder Cancer Institute, Brady Urological
Institute, Johns Hopkins Hospital, Baltimore,
Maryland, USA

DUNIA KHALED, MD
Clinical Instructor, Department of Urology, The
University of Kansas Medical Center, Kansas
City, Kansas, USA

BADRINATH R. KONETY, MD, MBA, FACS
Professor and Dougherty Family Chair in
Urologic Oncology, Department of Urology,
Vice Dean for Clinical Affairs, University of
Minnesota Medical School, Chief Executive
Officer, University of Minnesota Physicians,

Chief Clinical Officer, MHealth Fairview,
University of Minnesota, Minneapolis,
Minnesota, USA

WOJCIECH KRAJEWSKI, MD
Department of Urology and Oncological
Urology, Wrocław Medical University,
Wrocław, Poland

ROGER LI, MD
Department of Genitourinary Oncology, H. Lee
Moffitt Cancer Center, Tampa, Florida, USA

THOMAS A. LONGO, MD
Division of Urology, Duke University Medical
Center, Durham, North Carolina, USA

JAMES M. McKIERNAN, MD
John K. Lattimer Professor of Urology, Chair,
Columbia University Department of Urology,
Herbert Irving Pavilion, New York, New York,
USA

KIMBERLY A. McLAUGHLIN, BS, MS
Departments of Urology and Biochemistry,
Feinberg School of Medicine, Polsky Urologic
Cancer Institute, Robert H. Lurie
Comprehensive Cancer Center, Northwestern
University, Chicago, Illinois, USA

JOSHUA J. MEEKS, MD, PhD
Departments of Urology and Biochemistry,
Feinberg School of Medicine, Polsky Urologic
Cancer Institute, Robert H. Lurie
Comprehensive Cancer Center, Northwestern
University, Chicago, Illinois, USA

MAXWELL V. MENG, MD
Professor, Department of Urology, University
of California, San Francisco, San Francisco,
California, USA

VIKRAM M. NARAYAN, MD
Department of Urology, The University of
Texas MD Anderson Cancer Center, Houston,
Texas, USA

MICHAEL A. O'DONNELL, MD
Richard D Williams Professor of Urology,
Department of Urology, The University of Iowa
Hospitals and Clinics, Iowa City, Iowa, USA

JOAN PALOU, MD
Department of Urology, Fundacion Puigvert,
Autonomous University of Barcelona,
Barcelona, Spain

FRANCESCA PISANO, MD
Department of Urology, Fundacion Puigvert, Autonomous University of Barcelona, Barcelona, Spain

SIMA P. PORTEN, MD, MPH
Assistant Professor, Department of Urology, University of California, San Francisco, San Francisco, California, USA

SUBODH REGMI, MD
Department of Urology, University of Minnesota, Minneapolis, Minnesota, USA

NIRANJAN J. SATHIANATHEN, MD
Department of Urology, University of Minnesota, Minneapolis, Minnesota, USA; Department of Surgery, The University of Melbourne, Department of Cancer Surgery, Peter MacCallum Cancer Centre, Parkville, Victoria, Australia

WEI PHIN TAN, MD
Division of Urology, Duke University Medical Center, Durham, North Carolina, USA

JOHN TAYLOR, MD
Professor, Department of Urology, The University of Kansas Medical Center, Kansas City, Kansas, USA

Contents

High-risk non–muscle invasive bladder cancer is marked by frequent disease recurrences and risk of stage progression, contributing to high surveillance, treatment-related costs, and patient anxiety. Although the mainstay of high-risk non–muscle invasive bladder cancer clinical management remains transurethral resection followed by intravesical bacillus Calmette-Guérin (BCG), patients who develop BCG-unresponsive disease have few salvage options outside of a radical cystectomy with pelvic lymphadenectomy. This article provides a historical context relevant to the development of the BCG-unresponsive definition, an overview of current clinical trial expectations, and an introduction to this issue of Urologic Clinics.

The best predictors of response to intravesical immunotherapy are tumor grade and stage, tumor recurrence pattern, nomograms, panels of urinary cytokines, and fluorescent in situ hybridization patterns of urine cytology examinations. Future investigations on predictors of Bacillus Calmette-Guérin efficacy are needed to better select those patients who will really benefit from a conservative treatment. Hardly any of the proposed nomograms were designed to precisely predict the outcome of Bacillus Calmette-Guérin immunotherapy. A new nomogram for NMIBC recurrence and progression based on all non–muscle-invasive bladder cancer subgroups would include factors already proven in cancer prognosis and prediction.

Disease progression and recurrence are common among patients on Bacillus Calmette-Guérin (BCG) therapy, and options for bladder-preserving subsequent therapy remain limited. Ongoing efforts to develop better second-line bladder-sparing therapies rely on clinical trials of patients deemed to have failed management with BCG. This article describes historical definitions of BCG failure, as well as recent efforts to better delineate and refine the clinical criteria for identifying individual patients who will not benefit from further intravesical BCG therapy. It also reviews guidance from the most recent expert consensus panels and professional association guidelines regarding which patients should not receive additional BCG therapy.

UROLOGIC CLINICS OF NORTH AMERICA

FORTHCOMING ISSUES

May 2020
Male Infertility
James Hotaling, *Editor*

August 2020
Cancer Immunotherapy in Urology
Sujit S Nair and Ashutosh Tewari, *Editors*

November 2020
**Advanced and Metastatic Renal Cell
Carcinoma**
William C. Huang, Ezequiel Becher, *Editors*

RECENT ISSUES

November 2019
Considerations in Gender Reassignment
Lee C. Zhao, Rachel Bluebond-Langner, *Editors*

August 2019
Modern Management of Testicular Cancer
Sia Daneshmand, *Editor*

Preface

Intravesical Therapy for Nonmuscle Invasive Bladder Cancer: Twenty-First Century Edition

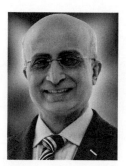

Badrinath R. Konety, MD, MBA, FACS
Editor

Since its approval in the 1980s, Bacillus Calmette-Guerin (BCG) has been the key agent for management of high-risk nonmuscle invasive bladder cancer (NMIBC). However, response rates are about 50%, and those who do respond do not always have a durable response. Repeat intravesical instillation with BCG and chemotherapy can salvage a small proportion of the nonresponders or those who recur later during the disease course. Patients deemed unresponsive to BCG or chemotherapy are particularly hard to treat and often require radical cystectomy. Options are limited to nonexistent for those who cannot tolerate cystectomy or do not want to proceed with cystectomy. Hence, there is an unmet need for the treatment of recalcitrant NMIBC. Repeated shortages of BCG have been commonplace, further limiting options even for the potentially BCG-responsive population. Several new agents and approaches have emerged to address this unmet need. The approaches being used range from use of modified BCG to gene therapy as well as combinations of intravesical chemotherapy. A completely new approach has been the systemic administration of checkpoint inhibitors to treat BCG-refractory disease. The field is exploding with new information and a plethora of trials and investigative methods to predict and assess response. Multidisciplinary management of bladder cancer is moving upstream and is no longer confined to muscle invasive bladder cancer or advanced disease. The excellent collection of articles in this issue authored by leaders in the field provides readers with an in-depth understanding of the current state of the field and what is yet to come.

Badrinath R. Konety, MD, MBA, FACS
Department of Urology
University of Minnesota
Medical School
University of Minnesota
C694, MMC 394
420 Delaware Street SE
Minneapolis, MN 55436, USA

E-mail address:
brkonety@umn.edu

https://doi.org/10.1016/j.ucl.2019.10.001

Bacillus Calmette-Guérin Salvage Therapy
Definitions and Context

Badrinath R. Konety, MD, MBA[a],*, Vikram M. Narayan, MD[b],
Colin P.N. Dinney, MD[b]

KEYWORDS

- BCG-unresponsive disease • Salvage intravesical therapy • Definitions of BCG-unresponsive
- BCG failure • Society of Urologic Oncology Clinical Trials Consortium
- High-risk non–muscle invasive bladder cancer

KEY POINTS

- High-risk non–muscle invasive bladder cancer (NMIBC) is aggressive and marked by frequent disease recurrences and risk of stage progression.
- Most patients with high-risk NMIBC eventually develop recurrent disease despite intravesical BCG therapy, and up to 35% of these patients die of their bladder cancer.
- BCG unresponsive disease is defined as disease in patients who have been treated with adequate BCG but who have recurrent disease, with adequate BCG defined as having received at least five of six induction instillations and at least two of three maintenance instillations.
- Salvage treatment options for patients who are cystectomy-ineligible and BCG-unresponsive are limited.
- Joint efforts by clinicians, industry partners, and the FDA have led to the establishment of well-defined trial registration objectives, with several resulting clinical trials planned and underway.

INTRODUCTION

Non–muscle invasive bladder cancer (NMIBC) remains a challenging disease to treat, with Ta, T1, and carcinoma in situ (CIS) stages comprising nearly 70% of all new diagnoses of bladder cancer.[1,2] High-risk NMIBC (defined by the American Urological Association/Society for Urologic Oncology [SUO] joint guidelines as T1 high-grade disease, any recurrent Ta high grade(HG) disease, Ta HG disease >3 cm or disease that is multifocal, presence of CIS, variant histology, lymphovascular invasion, high-grade prostatic urethral involvement, or prior bacillus Calmette-Guérin [BCG]

failure) is aggressive and marked by frequent disease recurrences and risk of stage progression, contributing to high surveillance, treatment-related costs, and patient anxiety.[3] Despite this, the mainstay of high-risk NMIBC clinical management remains transurethral resection of bladder tumor followed by intravesical instillations of BCG.

Estimates for the rates of disease recurrence following BCG therapy have ranged from 35% to 40%,[4–6] but true recurrence patterns are difficult to ascertain because of the different definitions of BCG failure and confounding conferred by patients receiving variable total doses of BCG. Nevertheless, it is reasonable to assume that

Disclosure Statement: C.P.N. Dinney: consultant for FKD Therapies Oy, Merck, NCI, and Jannsen; and research for Merck, NCI, and the University of Eastern Finland, Faculty of Health Sciences. The remaining authors have nothing to disclose.

[a] Department of Urology, University of Minnesota, 420 Delaware Street Southeast, MMC 394, Mayo B536, Minneapolis, MN 55455, USA; [b] Department of Urology, University of Texas MD Anderson Cancer Center, 1515 Holcombe Boulevard, Unit 1373, Houston, TX 77030, USA
* Corresponding author.
E-mail address: brkonety@umn.edu
Twitter: @VikramNarayan (V.M.N.)

Urol Clin N Am 47 (2020) 1–4
https://doi.org/10.1016/j.ucl.2019.09.002

most patients with NMIBC will eventually develop recurrent disease, and up to 35% of these patients will die of their bladder cancer.[7] The gold standard for BCG salvage therapy in high-risk NMIBC is to proceed with a radical cystectomy with bilateral pelvic lymphadenectomy, but this procedure is associated with significant morbidity and not all patients are appropriate surgical candidates. To date, the only alternative Food and Drug Administration (FDA)-approved therapy for BCG-refractory CIS is valrubicin, but this option is associated with a complete response (CR) rate of only 10% at 12 months.[8] There remains a significant unmet need for alternative effective salvage treatment options as second-line therapy for patients with NMIBC facing cystectomy.

DEFINING BACILLUS CALMETTE-GUÉRIN SALVAGE THERAPY

In 2012, the SUO along with representatives from the FDA met to discuss a registration strategy for trials being considered for the salvage treatment of patients with NMIBC. It is worth noting that at this point, patients who had "failed" BCG were referred to by terms that had vague or imprecise definitions, such as "BCG-refractory" or "BCG-resistant." The definition of these terms was based primarily on the treating physicians' interpretation of their patients' clinical status. At the Genitourinary Cancers Symposium in 2015, a task force helped clarify the disease state by formally establishing the term "BCG-unresponsive."[9] Patients who were classified as BCG-unresponsive were defined as those who had been treated with adequate BCG but had recurrent disease. Importantly, "adequate BCG" was defined as having received at least five of six induction instillations of BCG and at least two of three instillations of maintenance BCG.[10] The 2018 FDA statement on BCG-unresponsive NMIBC specifically defines BCG-unresponsive as patients who have:

- Persistent or recurrent CIS alone or with Ta/T1 disease within 12 months of adequate BCG therapy[10]
- Recurrent high-grade Ta/T1 disease within 6 months of adequate BCG therapy[10]
- T1 high-grade disease at the first evaluation following an induction course of BCG[10,11]

ADDRESSING THE PROBLEM: ESTABLISHING A TRIAL REGISTRATION STRATEGY

Of crucial concern was the lack of treatment options available for patients with BCG-unresponsive disease, and the dearth of clinical trials to address the unmet need in this space. Since 1959, only four agents had been approved for use in NMIBC. These included thiotepa for superficial papillary carcinoma of the urinary bladder (1959), doxorubicin (1974), BCG (1989) for CIS and prophylaxis of recurrent papillary tumors, and valrubicin (1998) for BCG-refractory CIS in patients for whom immediate cystectomy would be unacceptable.[12,13]

In 2012, under the aegis of the SUO Winter meeting in Bethesda, Maryland, a discussion took place among clinicians, industry partners, and the FDA to negotiate the terms for a registration strategy for BCG-unresponsive NMIBC. Among the issues raised included determining the most appropriate trial design type (single- vs double-arm design), clinically meaningful end points (recurrence-free survival or CR), and defining what constituted an appropriate patient mix to study (ie, a mixed population of Ta HG, T1, and CIS, vs cohorts of patients who only had CIS). The latter distinction was particularly important given that treatment of papillary bladder tumors is in essence adjuvant therapy following transurethral resection of bladder tumor, whereas treatment of CIS is classified as primary therapy. The SUO Clinical Trials Consortium/FDA meeting in November 2012 led to a consensus that ideal trials in this space should be comprised of a mixed population of HG tumors (CIS, Ta, and T1 tumors) with a minimum of 50% having some element of CIS. Single-arm trials were favored over two-arm trials, given that there currently exists no acceptable comparator treatment of patients who are BCG-unresponsive (aside from radical cystectomy, to which randomization would be challenging and not equivalent to medical intravesical therapy). Most on the panel considered 12 months to be an acceptable minimum duration for a clinically meaningful response. The SUO Clinical Trials Consortium bladder committee agreed on a 25% freedom from HG recurrence or CR as a meaningful clinical end point for success. A subsequent meeting between bladder cancer experts at the American Urological Association with the FDA in May 2013 provided further consensus in support of single-arm trial designs with a mixed population, acknowledging that the treatment intent for papillary tumors (adjuvant) and CIS (treatment) are distinct.[14] This panel initially recommended a goal CR of 40% to 50% at 6 months with a durable response rate of 30% at 18 to 24 months for CIS. Later these metrics were recognized as being overly ambitious, and the bar was lowered slightly to provide for an incremental but meaningful improvement over valrubicin.[15]

VALIDATING THE BACILLUS CALMETTE-GUÉRIN–UNRESPONSIVE DEFINITION AND THE HOPE FOR FUTURE THERAPEUTIC OPTIONS

The BCG-unresponsive definition was evaluated at the MD Anderson Cancer Center in a retrospective cohort study of 83 patients with NMIBC, 55 of whom were found to have satisfied the formal FDA definition of BCG-unresponsive disease, with the remaining 28 patients developing recurrence after induction therapy alone.[16] Although there were no differences between primary and recurrent tumor pathology of the two groups before or after receiving BCG, meeting the definition of BCG-unresponsive was independently predictive of worse cystectomy-free survival (hazard ratio, 3.85; 95% confidence interval, 1.49–10.0; $P = .006$).[16] Additionally, BCG-unresponsive patients had significantly worse high-grade recurrence free survival (hazard ratio, 6.25; 95% confidence interval, 2.27–16.67; $P<.001$). This study in part validated the futility of using currently available intravesical agents for patients who reached the BCG-unresponsive definition, and it further underscored the urgent need for new therapies in this area.[16] To this end, it is promising that there are at least eight ongoing clinical trials in the BCG-unresponsive space that are actively recruiting patients, including those considering systemic and intravesical treatment options. Additional trials are being planned at the time of this publication.

In summary, BCG-unresponsive disease remains a challenging disease to treat with limited therapeutic options aside from the gold-standard of radical cystectomy with pelvic lymphadenectomy. Participation in clinical trials in situations where it is safe and appropriate remain critical, particularly for patients who are not suitable candidates for surgery. Additionally, the dissemination, understanding, and correct use of BCG-unresponsive terminology is important, particularly when deciding on which patients may be best suited for clinical trial enrollment and in identifying patients for whom additional BCG therapy would be futile. This issue of *Urologic Clinics* seeks to highlight previous and ongoing efforts at developing alternative approaches to the management of intravesical treatment of high-risk BCG-unresponsive NMIBC, within the context of salvage therapy. The intermittent shortages of BCG that have affected our ability to treat this patient population makes the need for identification of alternatives even more acute. Current efforts suggest that several validated options could emerge for this challenging patient population in the near future.

REFERENCES

1. Sylvester RJ, van der Meijden APM, Oosterlinck W, et al. Predicting recurrence and progression in individual patients with stage Ta T1 bladder cancer using EORTC risk tables: a combined analysis of 2596 patients from seven EORTC trials. Eur Urol 2006; 49(3):466-5 [discussion: 475–77].
2. Fernandez-Gomez J, Madero R, Solsona E, et al. Predicting nonmuscle invasive bladder cancer recurrence and progression in patients treated with bacillus Calmette-Guérin: the CUETO scoring model. J Urol 2009;182(5):2195–203.
3. Chang SS, Boorjian SA, Chou R, et al. Diagnosis and treatment of non-muscle invasive bladder cancer: AUA/SUO guideline. J Urol 2016;196(4): 1021–9.
4. Sylvester RJ, van der Meijden APM, Witjes JA, et al. Bacillus Calmette-Guérin versus chemotherapy for the intravesical treatment of patients with carcinoma in situ of the bladder: a meta-analysis of the published results of randomized clinical trials. J Urol 2005;174(1):86–91 [discussion: 91–2].
5. Shelley M, Court JB, Kynaston H, et al. Intravesical bacillus Calmette-Guérin in Ta and T1 bladder cancer. Cochrane Database Syst Rev 2003;(4): CD001986.
6. Nepple KG, Lightfoot AJ, Rosevear HM, et al, Bladder Cancer Genitourinary Oncology Study Group. Bacillus Calmette-Guérin with or without interferon α-2b and megadose versus recommended daily allowance vitamins during induction and maintenance intravesical treatment of nonmuscle invasive bladder cancer. J Urol 2010;184(5):1915–9.
7. Raj GV, Herr H, Serio AM, et al. Treatment paradigm shift may improve survival of patients with high risk superficial bladder cancer. J Urol 2007;177(4): 1283–6 [discussion: 1286].
8. Dinney CPN, Greenberg RE, Steinberg GD. Intravesical valrubicin in patients with bladder carcinoma in situ and contraindication to or failure after bacillus Calmette-Guérin. Urol Oncol 2013;31(8):1635–42.
9. Lerner SP, Dinney C, Kamat A, et al. Clarification of bladder cancer disease states following treatment of patients with intravesical BCG. Bladder Cancer 2015;1(1):29–30.
10. Bacillus-Calmette-Guerin nunresponsive nonmuscle invasive bladder cancer:developing drugs and biologics for treatment guidance for industry. 2018. Available at: https://www.fda.gov/regulatory-information/search-fda-guidance-documents/bacillus-calmette-guerin-unresponsive-nonmuscle-invasive-bladder-cancer-developing-drugs and biologics for treatment guidance for industry. Accessed on 10.9.19.
11. Steinberg RL, Thomas LJ, Mott SL, et al. Bacillus Calmette-Guérin (BCG) treatment failures with non-muscle invasive bladder cancer: a data-driven

definition for BCG unresponsive disease. Bladder Cancer 2016;2(2):215–24.

12. Duplisea JJ, Mokkapati S, Plote D, et al. The development of interferon-based gene therapy for BCG unresponsive bladder cancer: from bench to bedside. World J Urol 2018. https://doi.org/10.1007/s00345-018-2553-7.

13. Logan C, Brown M, Hayne D. Intravesical therapies for bladder cancer: indications and limitations. BJU Int 2012;110:12–21.

14. Jarow JP, Lerner SP, Kluetz PG, et al. Clinical trial design for the development of new therapies for nonmuscle-invasive bladder cancer: report of a Food and Drug Administration and American Urological Association public workshop. Urology 2014;83(2):262–4.

15. Kamat AM, Sylvester RJ, Böhle A, et al. Definitions, end points, and clinical trial designs for nonmuscle-invasive bladder cancer: recommendations from the international bladder cancer group. J Clin Oncol 2016;34(16):1935–44.

16. Li R, Tabayoyong WB, Guo CC, et al. Prognostic implication of the United States Food and Drug Administration-defined BCG-unresponsive disease. Eur Urol 2019;75(1):8–10.

Salvage Therapies for Non–muscle-invasive Bladder Cancer: Who Will Respond to Bacillus Calmette-Guérin? Predictors and Nomograms

Óscar Rodríguez Faba, MD[a], Francesca Pisano, MD[a], Wojciech Krajewski, MD[b], Alberto Breda, MD[a], Joan Palou, MD[a],*

KEYWORDS

• Non-muscle invasive • Bladder cancer • BCG • Predictors • Nomograms • Recurrence

KEY POINTS

• The best predictors of response to Bacillus Calmette-Guérin are tumor grade and stage, recurrence pattern, nomograms, panels of urinary cytokines, and fluorescent in situ hybridization patterns of cytology.
• It has to be emphasized that hardly any of the proposed nomograms were designed to precisely predict the outcome of Bacillus Calmette-Guérin immunotherapy.
• A nomogram for non–muscle-invasive bladder cancer would be based on all non–muscle-invasive bladder cancer subgroups and would include factors that are already of proven value in prognosis and prediction.

INTRODUCTION

Among genitourinary tract tumors, urothelial bladder cancer represents the second most common diagnosis after prostate cancer. In Western countries, incidence rates have been increasing, with a prevalence of 500,000 cases per year in the United States.[1] At diagnosis, most such tumors are non–muscle-invasive bladder cancer (NMIBC). Among NMIBC, T1 high grade is considered to be a high-risk subgroup with an increased risk of progression that is sometimes characterized by the biological behavior of an invasive tumor. Its natural history suggests an unfavorable long-term outcome, as documented by early untreated series reporting a progression rate of 27% to 65% and a cancer-specific death rate of 34%.[1]

Bacillus Calmette-Guérin (BCG) is currently considered the gold standard conservative treatment for this kind of lesion,[2,3] but up to 30% of patients fail to respond initially and, of the responders, 74% eventually relapse. Patients with BCG failure are unlikely to respond to further

Disclosures: The authors declare that the development of the manuscript was not supported by an honorarium, a grant, or any other sources of support, including sponsorship or any material sources of support.
a Department of Urology, Fundacion Puigvert, carrer de Cartagena 340-350, 08025, Barcelona, Universitata Autonoma de Barcelona, Spain; b Department of Urology and Oncological Urology, Wroclaw Medical University, Ludwika Pasteura 1, 50-367 Wrocław, Poland
* Corresponding author.
E-mail address: jpalou@fundacio-puigvert.es

Urol Clin N Am 47 (2020) 5–13
https://doi.org/10.1016/j.ucl.2019.09.003
0094-0143/20/© 2019 Elsevier Inc. All rights reserved.

BCG therapy; moreover, delayed radical cystectomy is unlikely to be able to cure the disease.[3] A decrease in cancer-specific survival has been shown in patients with high-grade recurrence after BCG therapy who underwent radical cystectomy.[4] According to these findings, a delay in radical cystectomy seems to have a crucial role in the worsening of oncological outcomes.

PREDICTORS

Pathologic features have been the first factors used to predict the prognosis of bladder cancer. Based on these factors, prognostic models have been built, such as the European Organisation for Research and Treatment of Cancer (EORTC) and Club Urológico Español de Tratamiento Oncológico (CUETO) risk tables. Both of these models identify early recurrence and multiplicity as predictors of progression to muscle-invasive disease. Unfortunately, the available predictive models of recurrence and progression (EORTC) are unable to identify those patients who will not respond to intravesical immunotherapy with BCG.[2]

To date, a clear association between recurrent and multiple tumors and BCG response rate has not been found. In a population of 81 patients with stage T1G3 disease treated with BCG, neither multiplicity nor the presence of carcinoma in situ (CIS) was associated with the risk of failure of BCG treatment.[5] Similar results were previously highlighted by Cookson and Sarosdy.[6] According to these authors, tumor grade and stage, tumor multiplicity, and concurrent CIS before BCG did not predict tumor recurrence or progression. It is noteworthy that the role of concurrent CIS as a predictor of BCG response has been widely investigated. A number of studies have corroborated the relationship between the presence of CIS and a shorter recurrence- and progression-free survival in patients treated with BCG. In a series of 146 patients treated with BCG, the presence of CIS was the only predictor of progression, and consequently of poor BCG response, at multivariate analysis.[7]

Patient sex and age have also been investigated as potential predictors of response to BCG therapy. Even if female sex is associated with a worse prognosis, an investigation of a large series of 1021 consecutive patients treated with an induction course of BCG found no significant differences between men and women in terms of initial response, time to recurrence, or progression.[8] Because age could affect the integrity of the immune system, through which BCG acts, it has been supposed that older patients could

have an unsatisfactory response to BCG.[9] In confirmation of this hypothesis, a BCG plus interferon-alpha phase II study showed that patients older than 80 years had the poorest recurrence-free survival and that age over 80 years was independently associated with shorter recurrence-free survival.[9]

Even if the available risk tables are useful in the management of these groups of patients and in the prediction of risk of recurrence and progression, they are not equally accurate in predicting BCG response. Mainly owing to the lack of a standard BCG maintenance protocol among the patients used to elaborate the EORTC and CUETO risk tables, these models are unable to identify those patients who will not respond to intravesical immunotherapy with BCG.[2]

Recent studies have shown the role of lymphovascular invasion (LVI) and T1 substaging in predicting BCG response rates. According to Fukumoto and colleagues,[10] high-risk LVI-positive patients treated with BCG had a significantly lower progression-free survival rate compared with those without LVI (8.2% and 65.9%, respectively; $P = .015$). Similarly, patients with tumors deeply invading the lamina propria (HGT1b) showed a 3-fold increase in risk of progression, with lower response rates to BCG therapy.[11]

Biomarkers, the Immune System, and Cytokines

The host immune system plays a crucial role in the therapeutic effect of BCG.[12] Based on the mechanism of action of BCG, a number of studies have already been undertaken to evaluate the immunohistochemical pattern in tumor tissue as well as the serum and urine cytokine levels in patients with bladder cancer. It has been demonstrated that a higher level of leukocyturia after BCG induction is associated with improved response to BCG.[13] The mechanism of action of BCG seems to be partially related to the activity of antigen-presenting cells, like lymphocytes and natural killer cells.[14] Based on this observation, a number of studies were performed in immunocompetent patients, demonstrating an increase in the number of CD4$^+$ Th cells after BCG treatment and in the number of CD4$^+$ T cells (hazard ratio, 0.13; $P = .025$).[15] Similarly, Pichler and colleagues,[16] found that a decreased density of Th2-predominant CD4$^+$ T cells contributes to poor recurrence-free survival after BCG therapy. This interesting finding suggests a potential role of the tumor immune pattern in prediction of the therapeutic response to BCG, permitting individualized treatment.

Natural killer cells are considered a crucial element in the immune system activation induced by BCG treatment. Interactions between natural killer cells and tumor ligands have been suggested as potential predictors of BCG response. Yutkin and colleagues[17] evaluated tumor expression of natural cytotoxicity receptor ligands in specimens of transurethral resection of bladder tumor from patients with primary, non–muscle-invasive high-grade bladder cancer who were subsequently treated with BCG. According to their results, primary tumors from favorably responding patients expressed higher levels of ligand for all the tested proteins.

Another turning point in the understanding of BCG activity has been the recognition of the role of macrophages. In this field, 2 different studies found an association between higher numbers of tumor-infiltrating CD68[+] tumor-associated macrophages and higher recurrence rates after BCG and suggested that these cells are involved in the inflammatory circuit that promotes tumor progression.[18,19]

A number of biomarkers are currently under evaluation as predictors of response to BCG. Among them, the most promising seem to be RB, survivin, bcl-2, E-cadherin, ezrin, FGFR3, and Ki67.[20] To give an example, underexpression of RB and ezrin is a predictor of no response to BCG and increased risk of progression.[21] Conversely, the downregulation of FGFR3 predicts a good response.[22] Unfortunately, the available literature on biomarkers has several limitations, including nonstandard methods of measurement and lack of standardized cutoff and validation.

Urinary cytokines are one of the most promising prognostic markers in BC. They can be found in the urine within 1 to 4 weeks from the start of BCG treatment.[20] After gaining an increased understanding of their functions, cytokine profiles have been analyzed to assess the efficacy of BCG-induced cytotoxic response. IL-2 expression has been most extensively studied. When cytokine levels were evaluated in 39 patients receiving BCG for NMIBC or CIS, absence of urinary IL-2 during the BCG induction course and the first extended induction cycle (6 + 3 schedule) was found to correlate with time to recurrence ($P = .01$) and progression ($P = .01$). Similarly, Cai and colleagues[23] evaluated the potential role of the ratio between IL-6 and IL-10, comparing 72 patients affected by high-risk NMIBC with 49 controls. At multivariate analysis, IL-6/IL-10 ratio ($P<.003$) and the number of lesions ($P<.001$) were identified as independent predictors of probability of BCG response. Patients with an IL6/IL10 ratio of greater than 0.10 had a higher risk of recurrence and progression (**Table 1**).

Urinary fluorescent in situ hybridization (FISH) is a molecular cytogenetic test able to detect chromosomal abnormalities.[24] Thanks to its ability to anticipate tumor formation, FISH could be considered a valuable predictor of BCG response. Kamat and colleagues[25] evaluated the role of FISH in predicting BCG failure in a population of 126 patients treated with BCG. According to these authors, patients with a positive FISH result had a 58% risk of recurrence compared with 15% in patients with a negative result ($P<.001$) and a risk of progression of 25% compared with 7% in cases of negative FISH ($P<.013$).

Table 1
Predictive makers (BCG response)

Predictive Marker	Study	Determination
Ratio IL6/IL10 (23)	Prospective	Urine/ELISA
Leukocyturia (13) (during BCG treatment)	Prospective	Urine (counting)
CD4[+] (15)	Prospective	Tissue
Density Th2 (16)	Prospective	Tissue/IHC
Natural killer cells (17)	Retrospective	Tissue/IHC
Macrophages (18)	Prospective	IHC (density positive cells)
FGFR3 (22) (downregulation)	Prospective	Cell culture
FISH (24)	Prospective	Urine
Methylation (tumor suppressor genes)	Retrospective	Tissue
Cytokines (43) CyPRIT	Prospective	Urine
Ezrin (21)	Retrospective	Tissue/IHC

Abbreviation: IHC, immunohistochemistry.

Genomic Variant

Another theory has emerged from the idea that genomic variations affecting key genes implicated in BCG-induced inflammatory pathways could impact on BCG response rates. Leibovici and colleagues[26] observed that a variant genotype in IL-6 is associated with increased risk of recurrence with BCG. Their results supported the idea that inflammation gene polymorphisms are associated with a modified treatment response to BCG, with a consequent impact on survival.

Additional genes linked to outcomes following BCG treatment include those involved in detoxification (hGPX1), nucleotide exCISion repair and regulation of macrophage susceptibility to intracellular mycobacterial growth (NRAMP1).[20] Similarly, polymorphisms impairing cellular DNA damage repair have been associated with better outcomes after BCG treatment. In a population of 25 high-risk patients with NMIBC, selective next-generation sequencing was performed to compare the genomic profiles of cancers that responded to intravesical therapy and those that progressed to muscle-invasive disease.[27] This analysis found a significant decrease in total mutational burden to be associated with immunotherapy response. This association suggests that more advanced tumors have a decreased neoantigen burden and may explain the mechanism of BCG response in nonprogressors.

Methylation profiles have been examined in several panels of genes. Agundez and colleagues[28] assessed the role of the methylation of 25 tumor suppressor genes in predicting the prognosis in 91 patients with primary T1G3 tumors who were receiving BCG treatment. Their results confirmed the methylation status of tumor suppressor genes to be associated with the clinical outcome. The authors concluded that methylation status can be used to distinguish patients who will respond to BCG from those who will not.

Predicting Bacillus Calmette-Guérin Response in Carcinoma in Situ

Response to BCG is the result of complex molecular interactions between host and tumor. To date, not a single marker or test has been identified that can predict the precise response to BCG, either in CIS or in other NMIBC. Nonetheless, a combination of surrogate biomarkers and predictors of response has been studied in a heterogeneous population of NMIBC[20] and this combination could be cautiously extrapolated to CIS alone.

Clinicopathologic factors have been extensively studied by the EORTC[29] and CUETO groups.[30] Female sex, old age, high grade and stage, tumor multiplicity, early recurrence, and presence of CIS were identified as predictors of recurrence and progression of non–muscle-invasive tumors. One of the major drawbacks of the EORTC and CUETO studies is the disparity in BCG application and schedules. Moreover, the conclusions are related to poor tumor prognosis and caution must be exercised in assuming an association with BCG response itself, although it seems logical that a poor BCG response could be indicative of a worse outcome.

Urinary FISH (Urovysion, Abbot Molecular, Des Plaines, IL), a molecular cytogenetic test, can diagnose molecular failure after BCG and has been found capable of predicting subsequent tumor recurrence in the following 6 to 24 months.[31] In a recent meta-analysis including 6 studies and 442 patients, post-BCG FISH test had a sensitivity of 0.54 (95% confidence interval [CI], 0.38–0.69), a specificity of 0.84 (95% CI, 0.72–0.91) and an area under the curve of 0.78 (95% CI, 0.74–0.81) for predicting recurrences. Patients with a positive post-BCG FISH test were more likely to have recurrences during follow-up (hazard ratio, 3.95; 95% CI, 2.72–5.72).[32] No specific studies have been conducted exclusively for CIS. Many molecular biomarkers have been explored using immunohistochemistry. In a study conducted by Sato and colleagues[33] in 27 patients with CIS, tumors where analyzed before treatment and overexpression of pRb, p16, and p53 was found in 41%, 37%, and 48% of patients, respectively. pRb overexpression had a significant relationship with poor response to BCG therapy, but neither p16 nor p53 seemed to have a predictive value for initial BCG failure.

The lack of predictive value of p53 for CIS was also identified in other studies.[34,35] Other markers have been assessed for NMIBC (survivin, bcl-2, e-cadherin, ezrin, and Ki-67), but study heterogeneity at multiple levels makes response prediction unreliable when using only molecular biomarkers.

An indirect way of evaluating BCG-induced immunity is to measure the number and type of cells and cytokines involved in the immune response. This factor has been quantified in various samples (tumor, urine, and peripheral blood) and at different timings (before, during, and after treatment). Of all these tests, probably the one that stands out is determination of the polarity of lymphocytes and eosinophils in the tumor's microenvironment. The goal of BCG is to drive an immunomodulated response by changing immune cells' polarity from Th2 to Th1, and BCG has been found to have no effect if the microenvironment is already polarized to Th1 before treatment.[36] In this study, the proposed algorithm included 3 immunohistochemistry tests, 2 scores (eosinophil activity index and GATA-3[+]/T-bet[+] lymphocyte ratio) and a Th2 signature to assess response in patients with CIS. This tool was able to predict BCG response with 100% sensitivity and 80% specificity at the authors' proposed cutoff.

Other tools to assess immune response include evaluation of the presence of polymorphonuclear cells, because they are related to direct cytotoxicity through tumor necrosis factor-related apoptosis-inducing ligand.[37] Also, the dual role of macrophages has been assessed by 3 different studies, which concluded that presence of CD68[+] tumor-infiltrating macrophages predicts a higher number of recurrences after BCG.[18,19,38]

Antigen presentation-related molecules (heat shock protein 90, expression of major histocompatibility complex I and II) and signaling molecules (such as ICAM1) could also be an indirect sign of increased immune response. It remains unclear whether the presence of these molecules actually contributes in improving outcomes, because they are upregulated by the presence of interferon, which is always increased during BCG treatment.[39–42]

Urinary cytokines have also been widely assessed. Kamat and colleagues[43] created a nomogram (CyPRIT) using a panel of 9 inducible cytokines that seemed to have an accuracy of 85.5% (95% CI, 77.9%–93.1%) in predicting response. This diagnostic tool is currently under validation. Clinical immune response evaluation is an inconsistent way of drawing conclusions regarding the future response to BCG. Studies assessing adverse effects (eg, fever) have yielded controversial results, and although this could be related to a more energetic immunologic response, better outcomes in terms of recurrence or survival have not yet been proven.[44] Finally, genetic polymorphisms may have a role in BCG response. On the one hand, when impairing genes related to BCG-induced pathways (IL-6, IL-17, IL-2, tumor necrosis factor-α, MCP-1 and tumor necrosis factor-related apoptosis-inducing ligand receptor), they can be related to a worse response to BCG.[26,45] In contrast, when affecting DNA damage repair genes, they can contribute in increasing the tumor mutational burden, and subsequently to a better response to BCG and other new immunotherapies.[27,46] Further investigations are required to elucidate further the findings of all these studies.

Using the same NMBIC evaluation tools to predict response involves several shortcomings. First, CIS seems to have a different molecular pathway

in its origin compared with Ta/T1,[47] and extrapolation of results of the available tests is probably not completely reliable. Although no differences in BCG response between clusters were identified in this study, groups were small (n = 20) and the statistical power was insufficient to draw consistent conclusions. Moreover, most of the available studies have been applied in a heterogeneous population, mixing intermediate- and high-risk bladder cancer and also Ta/T1 with or without concomitant CIS. This makes it difficult to individualize conclusions for a subgroup of patients such as those with CIS alone.

Ongoing studies exploring CIS molecular origin, bladder cancer immunology, and tumor gene expression will help to resolve this puzzle and improve treatment choices and results.

NOMOGRAMS

Precise clinical risk assessment and identification of patients who will not benefit from conservative BCG immunotherapy is vital. Various scientific bodies have tried to facilitate this task by creating nomograms that are easy to use in everyday clinical practice. According to the latest update of the European Association of Urology guidelines, 2 nomograms are recommended for prediction of the NMIBC recurrence and progression risks. The first was constructed by the EORTC on the basis of data from 2596 patients diagnosed with TaT1 tumors and treated with adjuvant intravesical chemotherapy in 7 randomized EORTC trials. The scoring model included 6 factors (tumor stage, grade, focality and size, recurrence rate, and presence of CIS); a weight score was assessed for each factor to allow for the calculation of the total score and, finally, estimation of the risk using risk tables.[48]

The EORTC tables have been externally validated in several populations. Studies from Europe and Asia have shown the EORTC tables to be efficient in predicting recurrence and progression with high concordance indexes.[49–52] Also, a more recent study has validated the EORTC nomogram in 479 patients who underwent second (restaging) transurethral resection of bladder tumor. The authors found that especially in the intermediate-risk group, the model overestimates the risks of recurrence yet predicts tumor progression risk well.[53] However, it has to be stressed that the EORTC nomogram was mainly based on patients who did not receive BCG immunotherapy. Although the parameters used in the EORTC system are generally related to poor prognosis and reflect an inferior response to BCG, the reliability of the EORTC system in the BCG setting is limited.

Seo and colleagues[54] demonstrated the EORTC tables to be effective in predicting recurrence and progression in 251 patients treated with BCG, yet the predicted risks were higher than the actual number of events in the analyzed population. This observation has been confirmed in other studies.[55–57]

The second nomogram, recommended by the European Association of Urology, was created by CUETO for patients treated with BCG immunotherapy. It is based on an analysis of 1062 patients from four CUETO trials. Patients received 12 instillations over a 5- to 6-month period, and no immediate postoperative instillation or restaging transurethral resection of bladder was performed. The scoring system uses 7 prognostic factors: gender, age, recurrence rate, tumor stage, grade, focality, and CIS presence.[30]

Similar to the EORTC tables, the CUETO system has been externally validated by various authors. A recent study analyzing 414 T1G3 cancers showed that the CUETO scoring model underestimates the risk of tumor recurrence, but predicts well the risk of progression.[58] In another study conducted by Choi and colleagues,[52] similar underestimation for higher risk tumors was observed for recurrence, but not for progression (only 53% patients received BCG). In contrast, Xylinas and colleagues[57] showed, in a large multicenter population, that the CUETO tables overestimate the risks of recurrence and progression. However, only 11% of their patients were treated with BCG. In a recent study analyzing patients with intermediate- and high-risk NMIBC who received BCG with conventional maintenance it was found that the CUETO model underestimated the risk of recurrence in better risk patients and overestimated the risk of progression in poor risk patients.[29] It is worth mentioning that in this study the authors also analyzed prognostic factors for both cancer-specific survival and overall survival (stage and grade for cancer-specific survival and grade and age for overall survival).

It has to be highlighted that from the current perspective, neither the EORTC nor the CUETO model is free from flaws. When constructing both nomograms, only a relatively small number of T1G3/high-grade tumors, the most clinically important entity in salvage setting, were included. Similarly, few CIS cases were considered, limiting the models' value for both CIS prognosis and BCG response estimation. Neither system assessed prognostic factors known to impair BCG response, such as histologic variants and depth of submucosal or LVI, or analyzed the influence of restaging transurethral resection of bladder, the quality of the transurethral resection of bladder

or the value of immediate chemotherapy instillation. Number of BCG instillations, dosage, strain, or other factors that might theoretically be associated with BCG outcome were also not studied.[20]

In the recent literature, new nomograms aiming to meet current requirements are emerging. Ali-El-Dein and colleagues[59] constructed nomograms for tumor recurrence and progression, analyzing the data of 1019 patients treated mainly with adjuvant BCG immunotherapy. They incorporated tumor stage, focality, recurrence rate and method of adjuvant therapy in the recurrence nomogram and tumor grade and size, as well as method of adjuvant therapy, in the progression nomogram.

Kim and colleagues[60] composed a nomogram on the basis of 970 patients with primary NMIBC. LVI, variant histology (VH), gross hematuria, and history of upper tract urothelial carcinoma (UTUC) were incorporated in the mathematical model. The authors proved that gross hematuria and UTUCs are related to tumor recurrence and that UTUC and LVI are related to cancer progression. Similar to classic nomograms, this one is not free from imperfections. The analyzed population included a high number of T1LG tumors and UTUCs and a low number of CIS, LVIs, and VHs. Second, all the tumors were primary and only approximately 60% of patients were treated with some form of BCG immunotherapy.

Another new system was recently presented by D Andrea and colleagues.[61] On the basis of retrospective analysis of 1289 patients with T1G3 NMIBCs treated with more current regimens, the authors identified VH and LVI as associated with disease progression and created a nomogram to facilitate system usage. Although the study population was treated with various therapeutic regimens, CIS cases were excluded and once more the transurethral resection of bladder and restaging of transurethral resection of bladder tumor quality was not assessed, this nomogram strengthens the position of VH and LVI as prognostic and predictive factors. It has to be remembered that the majority of the available nomograms and mathematical models are designed for prediction of the risk of a clinical event (eg, recurrence, progression), and have not primarily been created for prediction of BCG immunotherapy response. From this it follows that although some factors incorporated in the nomograms are associated with the general poor prognosis of bladder cancer, this does not necessarily translate directly into the ability to predict a poor BCG response. A tool designed to predict BCG response was recently proposed by Kamat and colleagues.[43] In a prospective study of 125 patients, the authors measured cytokine levels in urine at various time points. Nine cytokines (IL2, IL-6, IL-8, IL-18, IL-1ra, tumor necrosis factor-related apoptosis-inducing ligand, interferon-γ, IL-12 [p70], and tumor necrosis factor-α) were found to have accuracy in predicting response to BCG immunotherapy in terms of recurrence. Despite the relatively low number of patients and the lack of staging and grading subanalyses, the proposed CyPRIT nomogram shows solid piece of evidence in.[43]

SUMMARY

Despite the number of investigations that have been conducted on this topic, the lack of a validated definition of BCG failure until the recent expert consensus on BCG-unresponsive disease has made it difficult to interpret and compare the results of the available studies. Currently, the best predictors of response to intravesical immunotherapy are tumor grade and stage, tumor recurrence pattern, nomograms such as the EORTC and CUETO tables, panels of urinary cytokines, and FISH patterns of urine cytology examinations. Future investigations on predictors of BCG efficacy are needed to better select those patients who will really benefit from a conservative treatment. It has to be emphasized that hardly any of the proposed nomograms were designed to precisely predict the outcome of BCG immunotherapy. Ideally, a new nomogram for NMIBC recurrence and progression (and cancer-specific mortality) would be based on all NMIBC subgroups treated with modern schedules and would include factors that are already of proven value in cancer prognosis and prediction. This is particularly important in high and very high-risk patients, as well as in the salvage setting.

REFERENCES

1. Jemal A, Siegel R, Ward E, et al. Cancer statistics, 2006. CA Cancer J Clin 2006;56:106–30.
2. Nieder AM, Brausi M, Lamm D, et al. Management of stage T1 tumors of the bladder: international Consensus Panel. Urology 2005;66:108–25.
3. Babjuk M, Bohle A, Burger M, et al. EAU guidelines on non-muscle-invasive urothelial carcinoma of the bladder: update 2016. Eur Urol 2017;71:447–61.
4. Kulkarni GS, Hakenberg OW, Gschwend JE, et al. An updated critical analysis of the treatment strategy for newly diagnosed high-grade T1 (previously T1G3) bladder cancer. Eur Urol 2010;57:60–70.
5. Pansadoro V, Emiliozzi P, de Paula F, et al. Long-term follow-up of G3T1 transitional cell carcinoma of the bladder treated with intravesical Bacille Calmette-Guerin: 18-year experience. Urology 2002;59:227–31.
6. Cookson MS, Sarosdy MF. Management of stage T1 superficial bladder cancer with intravesical bacillus Calmette-Guerin therapy. J Urol 1992;148:797–801.
7. Takashi M, Wakai K, Hattori T, et al. Evaluation of multiple recurrence events in superficial bladder cancer patients treated with intravesical bacillus Calmette-Guerin therapy using the Andersen-Gill's model. Int Urol Nephrol 2002;34:329–34.
8. Boorjian SA, Zhu F, Herr HW. The effect of gender on response to bacillus Calmette-Guerin therapy for patients with non-muscle-invasive urothelial carcinoma of the bladder. BJU Int 2010;106:357–61.
9. Joudi FN, Smith BJ, O'Donnell MA, et al. The impact of age on the response of patients with superficial bladder cancer to intravesical immunotherapy. J Urol 2006;175:1634–9 [discussion: 9–40].
10. Fukumoto K, Kikuchi E, Mikami S, et al. Lymphovascular invasion status at transurethral resection of bladder tumors may predict subsequent poor response of T1 tumors to bacillus Calmette-Guerin. BMC Urol 2016;16:5.
11. Orsola A, Werner L, de Torres I, et al. Reexamining treatment of high-grade T1 bladder cancer according to depth of lamina propria invasion: a prospective trial of 200 patients. Br J Cancer 2015;112:468–74.
12. van Rhijn BW, Liu L, Vis AN, et al. Prognostic value of molecular markers, sub-stage and European Organisation for the Research and Treatment of Cancer risk scores in primary T1 bladder cancer. BJU Int 2012;110:1169–76.
13. Saint F, Patard JJ, Irani J, et al. Leukocyturia as a predictor of tolerance and efficacy of intravesical BCG maintenance therapy for superficial bladder cancer. Urology 2001;57:617–21 [discussion: 21–2].
14. Ratliff TL, Palmer JO, McGarr JA, et al. Intravesical Bacillus Calmette-Guerin therapy for murine bladder tumors: initiation of the response by fibronectin-mediated attachment of Bacillus Calmette-Guerin. Cancer Res 1987;47:1762–6.
15. Bohle A, Gerdes J, Ulmer AJ, et al. Effects of local bacillus Calmette-Guerin therapy in patients with bladder carcinoma on immunocompetent cells of the bladder wall. J Urol 1990;144:53–8.
16. Pichler R, Fritz J, Zavadil C, et al. Tumor-infiltrating immune cell subpopulations influence the oncologic outcome after intravesical Bacillus Calmette-Guerin therapy in bladder cancer. Oncotarget 2016;7:39916–30.
17. Yutkin V, Pode D, Pikarsky E, et al. The expression level of ligands for natural killer cell receptors predicts response to bacillus Calmette-Guerin therapy: a pilot study. J Urol 2007;178:2660–4.

18. Ayari C, LaRue H, Hovington H, et al. Bladder tumor infiltrating mature dendritic cells and macrophages as predictors of response to bacillus Calmette-Guerin immunotherapy. Eur Urol 2009;55:1386–95.

19. Takayama H, Nishimura K, Tsujimura A, et al. Increased infiltration of tumor associated macrophages is associated with poor prognosis of bladder carcinoma in situ after intravesical bacillus Calmette-Guerin instillation. J Urol 2009;181:1894–900.

20. Kamat AM, Li R, O'Donnell MA, et al. Predicting response to intravesical Bacillus Calmette-Guerin immunotherapy: are we there yet? a systematic review. Eur Urol 2018;73:738–48.

21. Palou J, Algaba F, Vera I, et al. Protein expression patterns of ezrin are predictors of progression in T1G3 bladder tumours treated with nonmaintenance bacillus Calmette-Guerin. Eur Urol 2009;56:829–36.

22. Langle YV, Belgorosky D, Prack McCormick B, et al. FGFR3 down-regulation is involved in Bacillus Calmette-Guerin induced bladder tumor growth inhibition. J Urol 2016;195:188–97.

23. Cai T, Nesi G, Mazzoli S, et al. Prediction of response to bacillus Calmette-Guerin treatment in non-muscle invasive bladder cancer patients through interleukin-6 and interleukin-10 ratio. Exp Ther Med 2012;4:459–64.

24. Yoder BJ, Skacel M, Hedgepeth R, et al. Reflex UroVysion testing of bladder cancer surveillance patients with equivocal or negative urine cytology: a prospective study with focus on the natural history of anticipatory positive findings. Am J Clin Pathol 2007;127:295–301.

25. Kamat AM, Dickstein RJ, Messetti F, et al. Use of fluorescence in situ hybridization to predict response to bacillus Calmette-Guerin therapy for bladder cancer: results of a prospective trial. J Urol 2012;187:862–7.

26. Leibovici D, Grossman HB, Dinney CP, et al. Polymorphisms in inflammation genes and bladder cancer: from initiation to recurrence, progression, and survival. J Clin Oncol 2005;23:5746–56.

27. Meeks JJ, Carneiro BA, Pai SG, et al. Genomic characterization of high-risk non-muscle invasive bladder cancer. Oncotarget 2016;7:75176–84.

28. Agundez M, Grau L, Palou J, et al. Evaluation of the methylation status of tumour suppressor genes for predicting bacillus Calmette-Guerin response in patients with T1G3 high-risk bladder tumours. Eur Urol 2011;60:131–40.

29. Cambier S, Sylvester RJ, Collette L, et al. EORTC nomograms and risk groups for predicting recurrence, progression, and disease-specific and overall survival in non-muscle-invasive Stage Ta-T1 urothelial bladder cancer patients treated with 1-3 years of maintenance Bacillus Calmette-Guerin. Eur Urol 2016;69:60–9.

30. Fernandez-Gomez J, Madero R, Solsona E, et al. Predicting nonmuscle invasive bladder cancer recurrence and progression in patients treated with bacillus Calmette-Guerin: the CUETO scoring model. J Urol 2009;182:2195–203.

31. Kamat AM, Willis DL, Dickstein RJ, et al. Novel fluorescence in situ hybridization-based definition of Bacille Calmette-Guerin (BCG) failure for use in enhancing recruitment into clinical trials of intravesical therapies. BJU Int 2016;117:754–60.

32. Bao Y, Tu X, Chang T, et al. The role of fluorescence in situ hybridization to predict patient response to intravesical Bacillus Calmette-Guerin therapy for bladder cancer: a diagnostic meta-analysis and systematic review. Medicine (Baltimore) 2018;97:e12227.

33. Sato M, Yanai H, Morito T, et al. Association between the expression pattern of p16, pRb and p53 and the response to intravesical bacillus Calmette-Guerin therapy in patients with urothelial carcinoma in situ of the urinary bladder. Pathol Int 2011;61:456–60.

34. Ick K, Schultz M, Stout P, et al. Significance of p53 overexpression in urinary bladder transitional cell carcinoma in situ before and after bacillus Calmette-Guerin treatment. Urology 1997;49:541–6 [discussion: 6–7].

35. Shariat SF, Kim J, Raptidis G, et al. Association of p53 and p21 expression with clinical outcome in patients with carcinoma in situ of the urinary bladder. Urology 2003;61:1140–5.

36. Nunez-Nateras R, Castle EP, Protheroe CA, et al. Predicting response to bacillus Calmette-Guerin (BCG) in patients with carcinoma in situ of the bladder. Urol Oncol 2014;32:45.e23-30.

37. Ludwig AT, Moore JM, Luo Y, et al. Tumor necrosis factor-related apoptosis-inducing ligand: a novel mechanism for Bacillus Calmette-Guerin-induced antitumor activity. Cancer Res 2004;64:3386–90.

38. Ajili F, Kourda N, Darouiche A, et al. Prognostic value of tumor-associated macrophages count in human non-muscle-invasive bladder cancer treated by BCG immunotherapy. Ultrastruct Pathol 2013;37:56–61.

39. Lebret T, Watson RW, Molinie V, et al. HSP90 expression: a new predictive factor for BCG response in stage Ta-T1 grade 3 bladder tumours. Eur Urol 2007;51:161–6 [discussion: 6–7].

40. Videira PA, Calais FM, Correia M, et al. Efficacy of Bacille Calmette-Guerin immunotherapy predicted by expression of antigen-presenting molecules and chemokines. Urology 2009;74:944–50.

41. Jackson AM, Alexandroff AB, McIntyre M, et al. Induction of ICAM 1 expression on bladder tumours by BCG immunotherapy. J Clin Pathol 1994;47:309–12.

42. Prescott S, James K, Hargreave TB, et al. Intravesical Evans strain BCG therapy: quantitative

immunohistochemical analysis of the immune response within the bladder wall. J Urol 1992;147: 1636–42.

43. Kamat AM, Briggman J, Urbauer DL, et al. Cytokine panel for response to intravesical therapy (CyPRIT): nomogram of changes in urinary cytokine levels predicts patient response to Bacillus Calmette-Guerin. Eur Urol 2016;69:197–200.

44. Sylvester RJ, van der Meijden AP, Oosterlinck W, et al. The side effects of Bacillus Calmette-Guerin in the treatment of Ta T1 bladder cancer do not predict its efficacy: results from a European Organisation for Research and Treatment of Cancer Genito-Urinary Group Phase III trial. Eur Urol 2003;44: 423–8.

45. Lima L, Oliveira D, Ferreira JA, et al. The role of functional polymorphisms in immune response genes as biomarkers of Bacille Calmette-Guerin (BCG) immunotherapy outcome in bladder cancer: establishment of a predictive profile in a Southern Europe population. BJU Int 2015;116:753–63.

46. Gu J, Zhao H, Dinney CP, et al. Nucleotide excision repair gene polymorphisms and recurrence after treatment for superficial bladder cancer. Clin Cancer Res 2005;11:1408–15.

47. Hedegaard J, Lamy P, Nordentoft I, et al. Comprehensive transcriptional analysis of early-stage urothelial carcinoma. Cancer Cell 2016;30:27–42.

48. Sylvester RJ, van der Meijden AP, Oosterlinck W, et al. Predicting recurrence and progression in individual patients with stage Ta T1 bladder cancer using EORTC risk tables: a combined analysis of 2596 patients from seven EORTC trials. Eur Urol 2006;49: 475–7 [discussion: 75–7].

49. Hernandez V, De La Pena E, Martin MD, et al. External validation and applicability of the EORTC risk tables for non-muscle-invasive bladder cancer. World J Urol 2011;29:409–14.

50. Xu T, Zhu Z, Zhang X, et al. Predicting recurrence and progression in Chinese patients with nonmuscle-invasive bladder cancer using EORTC and CUETO scoring models. Urology 2013;82:387–93.

51. Ding W, Chen Z, Gou Y, et al. Are EORTC risk tables suitable for Chinese patients with non-muscle-invasive bladder cancer? Cancer Epidemiol 2014; 38:157–61.

52. Choi SY, Ryu JH, Chang IH, et al. Predicting recurrence and progression of non-muscle-invasive bladder cancer in Korean patients: a comparison of the EORTC and CUETO models. Korean J Urol 2014;55:643–9.

53. Zhang G, Steinbach D, Grimm MO, et al. Utility of the EORTC risk tables and CUETO scoring model for predicting recurrence and progression in non-muscle- invasive bladder cancer patients treated with routine second transurethral resection. World J Urol 2019. https://doi.org/10.1007/s00345-019-02681-2. [Epub ahead of print].

54. Seo KW, Kim BH, Park CH, et al. The efficacy of the EORTC scoring system and risk tables for the prediction of recurrence and progression of non-muscle-invasive bladder cancer after intravesical Bacillus Calmette-Guerin instillation. Korean J Urol 2010;51:165–70.

55. Altieri VM, Castellucci R, Palumbo P, et al. Recurrence and progression in non-muscle-invasive bladder cancer using EORTC risk tables. Urol Int 2012;89:61–6.

56. Kohjimoto Y, Kusumoto H, Nishizawa S, et al. External validation of European Organization for Research and Treatment of Cancer and Spanish Urological Club for Oncological Treatment scoring models to predict recurrence and progression in Japanese patients with non-muscle invasive bladder cancer treated with bacillus Calmette-Guerin. Int J Urol 2014;21:1201–7.

57. Xylinas E, Kent M, Kluth L, et al. Accuracy of the EORTC risk tables and of the CUETO scoring model to predict outcomes in non-muscle-invasive urothelial carcinoma of the bladder. Br J Cancer 2013; 109:1460–6.

58. Krajewski W, Rodriguez-Faba O, Breda A, et al. Validation of the CUETO scoring model for predicting recurrence and progression in T1G3 urothelial carcinoma of the bladder. Actas Urol Esp 2019;43(8): 445–51.

59. Ali-El-Dein B, Sooriakumaran P, Trinh QD, et al. Construction of predictive models for recurrence and progression in >1000 patients with non-muscle-invasive bladder cancer (NMIBC) from a single centre. BJU Int 2013;111:E331–41.

60. Kim HS, Jeong CW, Kwak C, et al. Novel nomograms to predict recurrence and progression in primary non-muscle-invasive bladder cancer: validation of predictive efficacy in comparison with European Organization of Research and Treatment of Cancer scoring system. World J Urol 2019;37(9): 1867–77.

61. D Andrea D, Abufaraj M, Susani M, et al. Accurate prediction of progression to muscle-invasive disease in patients with pT1G3 bladder cancer: a clinical decision-making tool. Urol Oncol 2018;36:239. e1-7.

Identification of Candidates for Salvage Therapy
The Past, Present, and Future of Defining Bacillus Calmette-Guérin Failure

Russell E.N. Becker, MD, PhD*, Max R. Kates, MD,
Trinity J. Bivalacqua, MD, PhD

KEYWORDS

- Bladder cancer • Nonmuscle-invasive bladder cancer • Intravesical therapy
- *Bacillus Calmette-Guérin* failure • *Bacillus Calmette-Guérin* unresponsive

KEY POINTS

- *Bacillus Calmette-Guérin* (BCG) failure is prevalent, and optimal management is unclear.
- Defining which patients will not benefit from further BCG therapy remains a significant challenge.
- High-quality primary evidence is limited, but expert panel consensus statements and professional association guidelines provide insight on best practices for management of patients with BCG failure.
- Radical cystectomy remains the gold standard of care for nonmuscle-invasive bladder cancer patients with BCG failure.
- Efforts to develop and improve alternative therapies are ongoing.

INTRODUCTION

For decades, intravesical instillation therapy with the attenuated mycobacterial strain *Bacillus Calmette-Guérin* (BCG) has been a mainstay of treatment for patients with intermediate- and high-risk nonmuscle-invasive bladder cancer (NMIBC).[1–3] However, disease progression and recurrence are common among patients on appropriate BCG therapy, and options for bladder-preserving subsequent therapy remain limited. Ongoing efforts to develop better second-line bladder-sparing therapies rely on clinical trials of patients deemed to have failed management with BCG. Both the design of these studies and critical interpretation of their results require the use of consistent definitions of BCG failure. Furthermore, these definitions serve a critical role in clarifying the clinical threshold for switching therapeutic strategies for a given patient. Proper definitions of BCG failure must therefore also be rational, systematic, and data-driven, to ensure that patients across all points along the BCG treatment and response spectrum receive optimal management.[4,5] Further complicating this challenge is the fact that accurate risk stratification in such patients must be dynamic, taking into account not only the parameters of a patient's disease at the time of initial diagnosis such as stage and grade, but also his or her individual treatment history,

Disclosures: The authors have no financial or other conflicts of interest to disclose.
The James Buchanan Brady Urological Institute and Greenberg Bladder Cancer Institute, Johns Hopkins University School of Medicine, Baltimore, MD 21287, USA
* Corresponding author:
E-mail address: rbecker@jhmi.edu

Urol Clin N Am 47 (2020) 15–21
https://doi.org/10.1016/j.ucl.2019.09.004

recurrence timeline, and the parameters of any recurrent tumors.[6] This article describes historical definitions of BCG failure, as well as recent efforts to better delineate and refine the clinical criteria for identifying individual patients who will not benefit from further intravesical BCG therapy. The authors also review guidance from the most recent expert consensus panels and professional association guidelines regarding which patients should not receive additional BCG therapy.

BACILLUS CALMETTE-GUÉRIN IN BLADDER CANCER MANAGEMENT: A BRIEF HISTORY

The antitumor potential of mycobacteria and the body's inflammatory reaction to them grew out of early observations from an autopsy series published by Pearl in 1929, in which patients infected with tuberculosis were found to have lower rates of cancers.[7] The *Mycobacterium bovis* strain *Bacillus Calmette-Guérin* (BCG), isolated from a heifer in 1913 and attenuated by serial passaging on glycerin-ox-bile, was already in widespread use in Europe as a vaccine against tuberculosis, and offered a more tenable mycobacterial model for capturing these desirable properties.[8] Several groups showed promising evidence of antitumor activity conferred by BCG injection therapy in murine models using transplanted tumors or tumor cell lines, and demonstrated the importance of close contact between BCG and the tumor in achieving these effects.[9–12]

The modern standard of adjuvant intravesical BCG following transurethral resection of bladder tumors (TURBT) was first described by Morales and colleagues[1] in 1976, in a retrospective series of 10 patients who received paired intravesical instillations and intradermal injections with the mycobacteria. The authors describe weekly dosing with a combination of intradermal and intravesical therapy for a total course of 6 weeks, and reported no tumor recurrences in limited follow-up. A short time later in 1982, a larger randomized controlled trial of 57 patients receiving either TURBT alone or TURBT with intravesical and intradermal BCG instillations showed a significant reduction in tumor recurrence (21% vs 50%, P=.027) with the addition of BCG adjuvant therapy.[12] Additional randomized trials demonstrated superior disease control with BCG when compared against existing adjuvant intravesical therapies: thiotepa and doxorubicin.[13,14] In 1990, BCG was approved by the US Food and Drug Administration (FDA) for the treatment of superficial bladder cancer. However, with this tremendous advance in therapy for NMIBC came a new set of problems in

determining how best to manage patients who did not respond. Indeed, BCG nonresponders were described in the literature as early as 1986.[15]

HISTORICAL DEFINITIONS OF BACILLUS CALMETTE-GUÉRIN FAILURE

With published rates of tumor recurrence and/or progression in the range of 30% to 50%, there are clearly many patients who do not exhibit the desired degree of antitumor response to intravesical BCG therapy. However, it has proven difficult for the field to agree upon a rigorous evidence-based and uniform set of criteria to identify those patients who will not benefit from further BCG therapy, and should therefore be advanced to alternative management strategies (Table 1). It is generally agreed that radical cystectomy is the current standard of care for such patients, but with its invasiveness and high rates of postoperative morbidity, this can be a difficult choice to justify for many patients and providers. As highlighted throughout this issue, efforts to develop novel salvage therapies for this difficult-to-manage patient population are ongoing.

The first modern attempt to rigorously define the patient population who would not benefit from further intravesical BCG therapy was published by Herr and Dalbagni in 2003.[16] The authors retrospectively reanalyzed data from a 1987 study randomizing patients to receive either induction BCG alone (6 weeks) or induction BCG plus an early iteration of maintenance BCG (monthly for 2 years). All patients had repeat TURBT at 3 months and 6 months. This early iteration of maintenance BCG showed no beneficial effect in its population. The authors found that tumor status at the 6-month evaluation, but not at the 3-month evaluation, was highly predictive of the overall 2-year recurrence-free rate (3-month tumor status hazard ratio [HR] 1.51, P=.24; 6-month tumor status HR 9.18, P=.001). Their work helped to establish the timing of tumor recurrence as an important indicator of BCG responsiveness, and hinted at the existence of an early (3-month) time window in which persistent tumors may still respond favorably to further BCG therapy, a finding further supported by several groups reporting durable response rates of 50% to 60% to a second induction course of BCG for persistent tumors seen after a single induction course.[15,17,18] In contrast, further attempts at BCG reinduction after failing 2 induction courses have been repeatedly shown to have limited or no added benefit.[19,20] Taken together, these data provide the foundation for one of the most widely accepted criteria for

Table 1
Professional association and consensus statement criteria for abandoning further *Bacillus Calmette-Guérin* therapy

GU-ASCO (2015)[23]	AUA/SUO (2016)[2]	EAU (2017)[3]	FDA (2018)[24]	ICUD/SIU (2019)[28]
HG at 6 mo evaluation[a]	HG or CIS within 6 mo after adequate BCG[a]	HGTa or CIS at 3 mo and 6 mo evaluations	HG within 6 mo after adequate BCG[a]	HG or worsening disease after adequate BCG[a]
HGT1 after single induction course	HGT1 after single induction course	HGT1 at 3 mo evaluation	HGT1 after single induction course	Disease progression after single induction course
HG relapse within 6 mo of last BCG exposure[a]		HG relapse within 6 mo of last BCG exposure		High-risk relapse within 6 mo of last BCG exposure[a]
	High-risk relapse within 12 mo after adequate BCG[a]			High-risk relapse within 12 mo after adequate BCG[a]
		CIS relapse within 12 mo of last BCG exposure	CIS within 12 mo after adequate BCG[a]	
		New HG appearing anytime during BCG therapy		

[a] Requires that patient received adequate BCG therapy, generally defined as at least 5 of 6 doses of an initial induction course, plus either 2 of 3 doses of a maintenance course, or 2 of 6 doses of a second induction course.

defining patients unlikely to benefit from further BCG: those who have recurrent or persistent tumor present upon completion of 2 courses of BCG (typically at the 6-month timepoint from initial diagnosis). It is also worth noting that, depending on their tumor status after the first induction course, patients may receive either a second induction course (6 weekly doses) or a first maintenance course (3 weekly doses). These 2 populations have typically been grouped together in defining BCG responsiveness categories, although it remains possible that they may exhibit somewhat different underlying pathobiology.

Two years later, in 2005, an international group of authors issued a consensus guidance statement regarding the management of stage T1 bladder tumors, which included the first detailed description of a nomenclature system for classifying BCG nonresponders into several subcategories.[21] The authors postulate some of these subcategories that were once grouped together as BCG failure may in fact be optimally managed with further BCG, including some patients with late relapsing disease. However, the authors did not provide specific clinical decision-making criteria. Their subcategory definitions were echoed in a 2006 review, and include[22]

- BCG refractory: failure to achieve a disease-free state by 6 months after initial BCG therapy with either maintenance or retreatment at 3 months because of either persistent or rapidly recurrent disease, also includes any progression in stage, grade, or disease extent by 3 months after the first cycle of BCG that is nonimproving or worsening disease despite BCG
- BCG resistant: recurrence or persistence of disease at 3 months after induction cycle but of lesser degree, stage, or grade that subsequently is no longer present at 6 months from BCG retreatment with or without TUR (disease improves then resolves with further BCG)
- BCG relapsing: recurrence of disease after achieving a disease-free status by 6 months (ie, disease resolves after BCG then returns); relapse is further defined by time of recurrence: early (within 12 months), intermediate (12–24 months), late (>24 months); relapsing

disease while on active maintenance (within 3 months) may qualify as BCG refractory

- BCG intolerant: disease recurrence after a less than adequate course of therapy is applied because of a serious adverse event or symptomatic intolerance that mandates discontinuation of further BCG (ie, recurrent disease in setting of inadequate BCG treatment from drug toxicity)

This nomenclature system has largely persisted, with subtle alterations, and remains commonly utilized in the current literature. Notably, however, the original descriptions did not provide a comprehensive definition of a population of patients who should not receive further BCG. The first attempt to do so did not come until 2015, when an expert panel was convened at the Genitourinary Cancers Symposium (GU-ASCO) in Florida to help guide clinical trial design for patients with BCG-unresponsive NMIBC.[23] This group of authors provided a new definition for a category of patients to be known as "BCG unresponsive," "who have been treated with adequate BCG…and are unlikely to benefit from and should not receive further intravesical BCG." Specifically, the GU-ASCO group included the following patients in its BCG unresponsive definition: (1) new or persistent high-grade tumor present at or around 6 months after initiation of BCG therapy, (2) relapse with high-grade tumor within 6 months of last intravesical exposure to BCG despite an initial complete response, or (3) high-grade T1 tumor present at first evaluation following induction BCG alone (at least 5 of 6 doses). They further stipulate that patients qualifying under either (1) or (2) must have completed "adequate BCG therapy," defined as receiving at least 5 of 6 doses of an initial induction course, and at least 2 of 3 doses of a maintenance course. This was later broadened by others to also include patients who have received 5 of 6 doses of a first induction course followed by 2 of 6 doses of a second induction course, in order to accommodate the increasing practice of administering a second induction course of BCG to those with a partial response after their first induction course.[24]

Beginning in 2011, the International Bladder Cancer Group (IBCG) expert panel also published several consensus statements regarding management of NMIBC and clinical trial design in this patient population, and specifically addressing the issue of defining and managing BCG failure.[5,25–27] Panel members propose that an important distinction must be made between treatment failure (any recurrence or progression during therapy) and recurrence (reappearance of disease after completion of therapy). Echoing the position of the international consensus statement[21] from 2005, they posit that certain patients with recurrent disease appearing after completion of BCG therapy can often be successfully managed with additional intravesical therapy.[25]

The major focus of the IBCG, however, has been on providing recommendations for standardization of clinical trials in NMIBC.[26] They specify that the subcategories of BCG refractory, BCG relapsing, and BCG intolerant as defined by Nieder and colleagues[21] should be used. Furthermore, they reaffirmed the GU-ASCO 2015 consensus panel[23] definition of a group of BCG unresponsive patients, including all patients with BCG refractory disease, as well as those with BCG relapsing disease within 6 months of their last BCG exposure.[26,27] For this group of BCG unresponsive patients, they specify that additional BCG intravesical therapy is not a feasible option, and radical cystectomy is considered the only standard of care management option. Because placebo controls are considered unethical in this population, and radical cystectomy is a drastically more invasive option that cannot practicably be randomized, the IBCG proposes that single-arm studies or comparison against investigator-choice alternative therapies are appropriate for testing novel salvage therapies in the BCG unresponsive patient population.

In aggregate, these studies and consensus statements present a relatively consistent, if not completely unified, set of definitions for patients who should not receive further BCG therapy. Yet further refinements to the nomenclature and clinical criteria for BCG failure are ongoing. In 2016, Steinberg and colleagues[20] performed retrospective cohort analysis on a group of patients enrolled in a phase 2 trial of intravesical BCG (at one-third the standard dose) mixed with interferon (IFN)-α. They specifically examined those patients in the trial who had previously failed intravesical BCG, and evaluated potential risk factors for developing recurrence of either pure papillary disease or CIS. Although those patients who had previously received 2 or more courses of BCG were more likely to fail the BCG plus IFN treatment regimen regardless of whether they had papillary disease or CIS, the time to BCG failure appeared to confer different levels of risk for the different disease subtypes. Hazard ratios for failing the BCG plus IFN regimen were calculated, using as a reference those patients with a history of BCG treatment whose recurrent disease developed greater than 12 months after therapy initiation. For those with papillary disease, a prior BCG failure within 6 months conferred significantly increased risk of failure of BCG plus IFN (HR 1.82, *P*=.02), while failure at 6 to 12 months carried identical risk compared to those with a prior failure interval greater than 12 months (HR 1.00, *P*=1.00). By contrast, for patients with a history of CIS and BCG failure, a failure interval of either less than 6 months (HR 2.59, *P*<.01) or 6 to 12 months (HR 2.29, *P*=.04) conferred a significantly greater risk of failing the BCG plus IFN treatment regimen, suggesting that the recurrence interval has dramatically different implications for patients with pure papillary disease versus CIS. Taken together, these data indicate that a patient with a pure papillary recurrence at greater than 6 months may have disease characteristics similar to a BCG-naïve patient, whereas recurrent CIS at up to 12 months carries an elevated risk of failing any attempted further BCG therapy.

The most recent consensus statement addressing BCG failure was published in early 2019 by the International Consultation on Urologic Diseases (ICUD) and the Société Internationale d'Urologie (SIU) and reflects an international expert panel convened in 2017.[28] They utilize the GU-ASCO framework nomenclature, reaffirming that patients with BCG unresponsive disease (BCG refractory disease, plus those with early relapse within 6–9 months of last BCG exposure) should not receive further BCG, and should be offered radical cystectomy as the standard of care.

ASSOCIATION GUIDELINES

Professional society guidelines for the management of NMIBC devote significant attention to the definition and management of BCG failure (see **Table 1**). The AUA/SUO guideline on diagnosis and treatment of NMIBC was most recently updated in 2016, and recommends that no further BCG therapy be administered to patients who either (1) are intolerant of BCG or (2) have a documented recurrence on TURBT of high-grade nonmuscle invasive disease and/or CIS within 6 months of 2 induction courses of BCG or induction BCG plus maintenance.[2] The European Association of Urology (EAU) guidelines, most recently updated in 2017, are highly concordant but with a slightly more wide-ranging timeline for high-grade recurrence.[3] In the European guideline, unsuccessful BCG treatment is defined by the persistence of high-grade disease at 3 months or the appearance of new high-grade disease (in a patient who previously had only low-grade disease) at any time during therapy, or by the presence of CIS at both 3 and 6 months after the initiation of BCG therapy (noting that a second course of BCG for those with CIS present at

3 months can achieve a complete response in up to 50% of patients by 6 months). The NCCN guidelines for bladder cancer, most recently updated in 2019, do not provide specific criteria for defining BCG failure or subcategories.[29] They do not make specific management recommendations, but stipulate that for post-treatment recurrent NMIBC, providers should take into account individual risks for disease progression including tumor stage, grade, size, and number, and viable management strategies may include further BCG, alternative adjuvant therapies, and radical cystectomy.

The extended 12-month recurrence window for CIS as described by Steinberg and colleagues[20] was incorporated into a guidance statement issued by the US Food and Drug Administration (FDA) in 2018, targeted at standardizing the design of clinical trials for BCG-unresponsive NMIBC.[24] Among other specifications, they reaffirm that radical cystectomy is the standard of care for such patients, and that single-arm studies are acceptable in the BCG unresponsive disease state given the known likelihood of disease progression without therapy, impracticality of randomization to cystectomy, and lack of effective comparator therapies. They provide a strict definition of BCG unresponsive disease largely based on the framework of the GU-ASCO panel, which includes

> Patients with persistent or recurrent CIS alone or with recurrent Ta/T1 disease within 12 months of completion of adequate BCG therapy (defined as at least 5 of 6 doses of initial induction, plus at least 2 of 3 doses of a maintenance course or 2 of 6 doses of a second induction course)
> Recurrent high-grade Ta/T1 disease within 6 months of completion of adequate BCG therapy
> T1 high-grade disease at the first evaluation following an induction BCG course

Although the FDA guidance statement does not explicitly describe how to categorize recurrent disease arising in the context of additional ongoing BCG therapy (ie, maintenance therapy), it is generally accepted by the field that the 6- and 12-month timeframes used in the definitions are to be measured from the time of most recent BCG exposure.

FUTURE DIRECTIONS

As described throughout this issue, much remains to be determined in the optimal management of NMIBC and BCG failure. In particular, the authors recommend that future efforts should focus on improving the prognostic stratification and management of intermediate-risk NMIBC, as defined by AUA and EAU guidelines. This common disease category is a particular challenge for patients and providers alike, because of the large degree of heterogeneity and uncertainty in determining its optimal management. Novel biomarkers and prognostic tools will be particularly important in this group to better predict disease behavior and guide management. This is also an important patient population for the development of novel therapeutic strategies, although the high degree of heterogeneity within this group should be carefully considered and controlled for when designing studies. Another area of interest is to better elucidate the cellular and molecular mechanisms for the BCG antitumor response, including the concept of "priming," whereby early antigenic exposure may help train the body's immune system to mount a powerful antitumor response. Finally, even as development of new therapies continues, disruptions in the usable supply of BCG impose logistical constraints onto its use, further emphasizing the need for an expanded armamentarium against this common disease entity.

SUMMARY

Intravesical BCG therapy is the adjuvant treatment of choice and standard of care following thorough TURBT for intermediate- and high-risk NMIBC. However, rates of BCG failure remain high. Efforts to develop and improve alternative management strategies for NMIBC patients who fail BCG are ongoing, as highlighted throughout this issue. However, radical cystectomy, with high rates of perioperative morbidity, remains the accepted gold standard of care. Shortages of the BCG supply chain, such as the current shortage in the United States, further emphasize the need for viable alternative management strategies.

Accurate assessment of the risks of disease recurrence and progression in NMIBC patients requires careful consideration of multiple dynamic factors, including patient and tumor biology, as well as prior therapies received, with the timeline of therapeutic interventions and disease states playing a pivotal and complex role. Despite limited high-quality primary data, there is general consensus among expert panels and association guidelines in identifying those patients and tumors unlikely to respond to further BCG therapy. Future efforts must focus on further refinement and unification of precise, clinical evidence-based thresholds for

abandoning further BCG therapy, with the goal of minimizing the number of patients whose disease and treatment history place them in the uncertain gray area between receiving further BCG or progressing to alternative management strategies. Current evidence suggests that these thresholds may be markedly different for different stages and subtypes of NMIBC. If one is to provide optimal care for each patient with this challenging disease entity, further study is needed.

REFERENCES

1. Morales A, Eidinger D, Bruce AW. Intracavitary bacillus calmette-guerin in the treatment of superficial bladder tumors. J Urol 1976;116(2):180–3.
2. Chang SS, Boorjian SA, Chou R, et al. Diagnosis and treatment of non-muscle invasive bladder cancer: AUA/SUO guideline. J Urol 2016;196(4):1021–9.
3. Babjuk M, Böhle A, Burger M, et al. EAU guidelines on non-muscle-invasive urothelial carcinoma of the bladder: Update 2016. Eur Urol 2017;71(3):447–61.
4. Steinberg RL, Thomas LJ, O'Donnell MA. Bacillus calmette-guérin (BCG) treatment failures in non-muscle invasive bladder cancer: What truly constitutes unresponsive disease. Bladder Cancer 2015;1(2):105–16.
5. Lamm D, Persad R, Brausi M, et al. Defining progression in nonmuscle invasive bladder cancer: It is time for a new, standard definition. J Urol 2014;191(1):20–7.
6. McKiernan J. *Bacillus Calmette-Guérin* failure in non-muscle-invasive bladder cancer: One size does not fit all. Eur Urol 2016;70(5):786–7.
7. Pearl R. Cancer and tuberculosis. Am J Epidemiol 1929;9(1):97–159. Available at: https://academic.oup.com/aje/article/9/1/97/107352. Accessed April 25, 2019.
8. Petroff SA, Branch A. *Bacillus Calmette-Guérin* (B.C.G.) in prophylactic immunization in children : an analysis and critical review. Can Med Assoc J 1928;18(5):581–4.
9. Old LJ, Clarke DA, Benacerraf B. Effect of *Bacillus Calmette-Guerin* infection on transplanted tumours in the mouse. Nature 1959;184(Suppl 5):291–2.
10. Zbar B, Tanaka T. Immunotherapy of cancer: regression of tumors after intralesional injection of living *Mycobacterium bovis*. Science 1971;172(3980):271–3.
11. Zbar B, Bernstein ID, Bartlett GL, et al. Immunotherapy of cancer: regression of intradermal tumors and prevention of growth of lymph node metastases after intralesional injection of living *Mycobacterium bovis*. J Natl Cancer Inst 1972;49(1):119–30.
12. Lamm DL, Thor DE, Stogdill VD, et al. Bladder cancer immunotherapy. J Urol 1982;128(5):931–5.

13. Brosman SA. Experience with *Bacillus Calmette-Guerin* in patients with superficial bladder carcinoma. J Urol 1982;128(1):27–30.

14. Lamm DL, Blumenstein BA, Crawford ED, et al. A randomized trial of intravesical doxorubicin and immunotherapy with *Bacille Calmette-Guérin* for transitional-cell carcinoma of the bladder. N Engl J Med 1991;325(17):1205–9.

15. Haaff EO, Dresner SM, Ratliff TL, et al. Two courses of intravesical *Bacillus Calmette-Guerin* for transitional cell carcinoma of the bladder. J Urol 1986; 136(4):820–4.

16. Herr HW, Dalbagni G. Defining *Bacillus Calmette-Guerin* refractory superficial bladder tumors. J Urol 2003;169(5):1706–8.

17. Coplen DE, Marcus MD, Myers JA, et al. Long-term follow up of patients treated with 1 or 2, 6-week courses of intravesical *Bacillus Calmette-Guerin*: analysis of possible predictors of response free of tumor. J Urol 1990;144(3):652–7.

18. Kavoussi LR, Torrence RJ, Gillen DP, et al. Results of 6 weekly intravesical *Bacillus Calmette-Guerin* instillations on the treatment of superficial bladder tumors. J Urol 1988;139(5):935–40.

19. Catalona WJ, Hudson MA, Gillen DP, et al. Risks and benefits of repeated courses of intravesical *Bacillus Calmette-Guerin* therapy for superficial bladder cancer. J Urol 1987;137(2):220–4.

20. Steinberg RL, Thomas LJ, Mott SL, et al. *Bacillus Calmette-Guérin* (BCG) treatment failures with non-muscle invasive bladder cancer: a data-driven definition for BCG unresponsive disease. Bladder Cancer 2016;2(2):215–24.

21. Nieder AM, Brausi M, Lamm D, et al. Management of stage T1 tumors of the bladder: international consensus panel. Urology 2005;66(6 Suppl 1): 108–25.

22. O'Donnell MA, Boehle A. Treatment options for BCG failures. World J Urol 2006;24(5):481–7.

23. Lerner SP, Dinney C, Kamat A, et al. Clarification of bladder cancer disease states following treatment of patients with intravesical BCG. Bladder Cancer 2015;1(1):29–30.

24. United States Food and Drug Administration. BCG-unresponsive nonmuscle invasive bladder cancer: developing drugs and biologics for treatment. United States Food and Drug Administration; 2018 . Available at: https://www.fda.gov/media/101468/download.

25. Brausi M, Witjes JA, Lamm D, et al. A review of current guidelines and best practice recommendations for the management of nonmuscle invasive bladder cancer by the international bladder cancer group. J Urol 2011;186(6):2158–67.

26. Kamat AM, Sylvester RJ, Böhle A, et al. Definitions, end points, and clinical trial designs for non-muscle-invasive bladder cancer: recommendations from the international bladder cancer group. J Clin Oncol 2016;34(16):1935–44.

27. Kamat AM, Colombel M, Sundi D, et al. BCG-unresponsive non-muscle-invasive bladder cancer: recommendations from the IBCG. Nat Rev Urol 2017; 14(4):244–55. Available at: https://www.nature.com/articles/nrurol.2017.16. Accessed February 23, 2019.

28. Monteiro LL, Witjes JA, Agarwal PK, et al. ICUD-SIU international consultation on bladder cancer 2017: management of non-muscle invasive bladder cancer. World J Urol 2019;37(1):51–60.

29. National Comprehensive Cancer Network. NCCN clinical practice guidelines in oncology: bladder cancer (version 3.2019). National Comprehensive Cancer Network; 2019. Available at: https://www.nccn.org/professionals/physician_gls/pdf/bladder.pdf.

Predictors of Response to Intravesical Therapy

Roger Li, MD[a], Ashish M. Kamat, MD[b],*

KEYWORDS

- Bladder cancer • BCG • BCG-unresponsive disease • Immunotherapy • Intravesical therapy

KEY POINTS

- Tumor characteristics such as grade, stage, concomitant carcinoma in situ, and other molecular markers are likely prognostic of oncologic outcomes, rather than predictive of response to intravesical bacillus Calmette-Guérin (BCG).
- Host factors such as age, gender, genetic polymorphisms, and host microbiome may play crucial a role in the response to intravesical BCG.
- Additional predictors of response can be deduced from further elucidation of the mechanism of immunostimulation by intravesical BCG.

INTRODUCTION

It has been more than 4 decades since Morales and colleagues[1] first introduced the use of bacillus Calmette-Guérin (BCG) for non–muscle-invasive bladder cancer (NMIBC). Despite its reign as the most effective immunotherapy to date in urologic cancers, recurrence rates range between 32.6% and 42.1% and progression rates between 9.5% and 13.4%.[2,3] Progression clearly leads to compromised survival[4]; recurrent, nonprogressive disease is also problematic because of repeated procedures and intensive surveillance protocol. The lack of clinical tools to accurately predict response to therapy has hampered progress. Recent advances in the understanding of bladder cancer biology have provided a pathway to identifying early markers of response and of failure.

Although many investigators have focused on using intrinsic tumor characteristics to predict outcomes, because BCG renders its antineoplastic effects indirectly via stimulation of the immune system, host factors may also play a key role in treatment efficacy. In addition, accurate predictors

of responsiveness ultimately rely on the understanding of BCG's mechanism of action, which has been stubbornly difficult to elucidate. Nevertheless, several aspects of the BCG-elicited immunogenic reaction have been identified, measured, and linked to response. This article summarizes the published evidence on markers of response to intravesical immunotherapy with BCG.

TUMOR FACTORS

Two large studies by the Club Urologico Espano de Tratamiento Oncologico (CUETO) and European Organisation for Research and Treatment of Cancer (EORTC) groups attempted to link baseline clinicopathologic features to BCG response. In a cohort of 1062 patients, the CUETO group identified female gender, recurrent tumors, multiplicity, and the presence of carcinoma in situ (CIS) as predictors of recurrence, whereas recurrent tumors, high-grade tumors, T1 tumors, and recurrence on 3-month endoscopic examination were found to predict progression to muscle invasive bladder

Disclosures: None.
[a] Department of Genitourinary Oncology, H. Lee Moffitt Cancer Center, Tampa, FL, USA; [b] Department of Urology, The University of Texas MD Anderson Cancer Center, 1515 Holcombe Boulevard, Unit 1373, Houston, TX 77030, USA
* Corresponding author.
E-mail address: akamat@mdanderson.org

Urol Clin N Am 47 (2020) 23–33
https://doi.org/10.1016/j.ucl.2019.09.005

cancer (MIBC).[3] From these findings, a scoring system was constructed to categorize the patients into 4 risk groups for recurrence (C index, 0.64) and progression (C index, 0.69–0.70).[5]

In a similar study consisting of 1812 patients, the EORTC found that prior recurrence rate greater than 1 per year, tumor multiplicity (≥4 tumors), and tumor grade predicted early recurrence after BCG induction (C index, 0.65–0.67). Similarly, late recurrence was also predicted by prior recurrence rate greater than 1 per year and tumor multiplicity (C index, 0.56–0.59). In contrast, tumor grade and T stage were significant predictors of disease progression (C index, 0.64–0.72).[2] One notable difference between the 2 cohorts studied was the difference in the maintenance BCG schedule. Although the CUETO group used a nonstandard maintenance protocol of 6 fortnightly treatments after induction, the EORTC study was conducted in patients who received 1 to 3 years of maintenance therapy in accordance with the Southwest Oncology Group (SWOG) (6 + 3) protocol.[2] Nevertheless, it is noteworthy that these 2 large studies independently found prior recurrence and tumor multiplicity to be predictors for future recurrence, and high grade and stage to be predictors for progression after BCG treatment.

The association between high tumor grade and stage with subsequent disease progression following BCG treatment is likely a reflection of their poor prognostic value. Independent of treatment modality, progression rate in high-grade T1 bladder cancer was found to be 21%.[6] In addition, understaging is a well-described phenomenon in bladder cancer, occurring in up to 50% of patients with presumed non–muscle-invasive high-grade disease.[7] Although effective for NMIBC, BCG is thought to be futile against MIBC. Thus, treatment failure in a subset of patients with high-grade NMIBC may be a byproduct of understaging.

In addition, the presence of CIS has been extensively examined as a predictor of BCG failure. In 2 cohorts treated only with induction BCG, concomitant CIS was found to be a predictor of shorter progression-free survival (PFS) and cancer-specific survival (CSS).[8,9] The effect was especially pronounced in patients with T1 disease treated with induction BCG, in whom the presence of CIS led to a 58% progression rate to T2 disease or higher.[8] This finding was subsequently corroborated in a cohort treated with induction and maintenance therapy.[10]

Contrastingly, the association between prior recurrence and tumor multiplicity with response to BCG is more controversial, with different studies yielding divergent results.[11–14] However, many studies indicating no association were underpowered or did not use maintenance therapy according to current standards. A recent review by an expert panel deemed these tumor characteristics to be important for predicting treatment response.[15]

Aside from the traditional clinicopathologic features, expression levels of molecular biomarkers also correlate with response to therapy. Of these, p53, a cell cycle regulator, has been the most extensively studied. Several groups have linked immunohistochemistry (IHC) p53 overexpression to disease progression after intravesical BCG.[16–18] However, it is unknown whether p53 overexpression on IHC correlated with loss of function. In addition, variations in p53 quantification methods and arbitrary thresholds make it difficult to compare results across studies.[19] For instance, several different anti-p53 antibodies are commercially available. These antibodies differ with regard to the epitope each recognizes, and thus can lead to different results. Overall, it is generally thought that the available information does not justify the use of p53 in clinical decision making.[19]

A multitude of other molecules have been examined as potential predictors for BCG response, including cell cycle regulators (Retinoblastoma protein), apoptosis inhibitors (survivin, bcl-2), cell adhesion molecules (E-cadherin, ezrin), and markers of proliferation (Ki-67). However, these studies all have similar shortfalls to those investigating p53: inconsistent diagnostic standards, inadequate study populations, and the lack of validation. Given the immense phenotypic heterogeneity within bladder cancer as well as the complex mechanism of action of BCG, it is unlikely that single biomarkers can accurately predict treatment success.[15]

One analysis accounting for some of the genotypic heterogeneity in bladder cancer is the UroVysion fluorescence in situ hybridization (FISH) test, which detects increased copy numbers of chromosomes 3, 7, and 17, and loss of 9p21, all putative chromosomal abnormalities found in bladder cancer.[20] A positive FISH result after BCG induction confers increased risk of recurrence (3-fold to 5-fold) and progression (5-fold to 13-fold), depending on timing of FISH positivity.[21] By virtue of its ability to anticipate tumor formation, FISH is a valuable clinical tool for predicting failure after BCG. Because many patients who have a positive FISH test have no visible tumor at the time of assessment but subsequently develop recurrence in 6 to 24 months, this phenomenon has been dubbed molecular failure and such patients would be ideal candidates to enroll into clinical trials for combination immunotherapeutic agents.[22]

The use of next-generation sequencing for the comprehensive molecular characterization of bladder cancer has not only shed light on tumor biology but also provided clues for molecular mechanisms of treatment success and failure. With regard to chemotherapy for MIBC, therapy-driven clonal evolution leading to chemoresistance has been shown.[23] Furthermore, somatic mutations in DNA damage repair (DDR) genes also seem to confer cisplatin-based chemosensitivity,[24] and molecular subtyping of MIBC has been linked to different phenotypic responses after neoadjuvant chemotherapy.[25]

In NMIBC, polymorphisms impairing cellular DDR have also been associated with better outcomes after BCG.[26] This association is thought to stem from the higher mutational burden and neoantigen load, which ultimately provokes a stronger immunogenic response. In a recent study of patients with high-risk NMIBC, a higher total mutation burden was found in patients who responded to intravesical therapy compared with those who did not.[27] In contrast, initial efforts in NMIBC molecular subtyping did not correlate with BCG response.[28] However, others have identified ARID1A mutations to be significantly associated with an increased risk of recurrence after BCG treatment (hazard ratio, 3.14; $P = .002$).[29] Further elucidation of the NMIBC molecular landscape and refinement of classifications may lead to insights on tumor biology and therapeutic efficacy.

HOST FACTORS

From the CUETO study, female gender and age both emerged as poor prognosticators for BCG response.[3] Palou and colleagues[30] subsequently corroborated the higher recurrence and progression rates in women treated with BCG. The urinary cytokine profile observed in women after BCG treatment is different than that found in men.[31] Because stimulation through the androgen axis is implicated in the development and progression of bladder cancer,[32] it is conceivable that differences in the hormonal milieu may also play a role in the responsiveness to immunotherapy.

Poorer outcomes seen in elderly patients intuitively stem from a weaker BCG response caused by their waning immune systems.[3,33] At first glance, patients more than 80 years old had the poorest recurrence-free survival (RFS) in a subset analysis of the phase 2 combination BCG/interferon (IFN)-α trial.[33] In another study, although initial response rates were equivalent in patients more than and less than 70 years old, more older patients recurred on long-term follow-up.[12]

Analysis of the prospective EORTC 30911 study recapitulated the poor prognostic effect of age on RFS, PFS, and CSS in BCG-treated patients[34]; however, even in older patients (>70 yeas old), BCG was more effective than epirubicin. Thus, old age seems to be more prognostic than it is predictive, and applies to patients undergoing all intravesical therapies.

Besides age, other host factors potentially affecting the immunogenic response have recently been interrogated. Variant polymorphisms in genes encoding several cytokines (interleukin [IL]-6, IL-17, IL-2, and tumor necrosis factor [TNF]-α), chemokines (MCP-1) as well as effector molecules (TNF-related apoptosis-inducing ligand [TRAIL] receptor) were associated with increased recurrence after BCG.[35,36] Adding these genomic signatures to key clinicopathologic features, a risk score was constructed and shown to achieve an area under the curve of 82% for predicting treatment response.[36] In addition, genes involved in detoxification (hGPX1), nucleotide excision repair, and regulation of macrophage susceptibility to intracellular mycobacterial growth (NRMAP1) were also shown to be influential on BCG treatment outcomes.[15]

Polymorphisms impairing cellular DDR may lead to higher mutational burden and levels of neoantigens that ultimately provoke a stronger immune response following BCG. Both DDR polymorphisms and high mutational burden have been linked to response to intravesical BCG.[26,27] Overall, associations between gene polymorphisms and BCG response warrant further exploration. Moreover, because most such studies were performed in homogenous ethnic and/or geographic populations, whether these associations can be extended to the global population remains to be seen.

Emerging evidence suggests that the unique microbial ecosystems may profoundly affect response to different cancer treatments. In its simplest form, many members of the gastrointestinal microbiota are known to influence the metabolism, pharmacokinetics, and toxicity of drugs.[37] For instance, Mycoplasma hyorhinis can metabolize and inactivate the chemotherapy agent gemcitabine, leading to drug resistance.[38] Although the mechanism is not yet completely understood, the efficacy of immune checkpoint blockade is also influenced by the gastrointestinal microbiome.[39,40] In animal models, eradication of certain commensal organisms using antibiotics led to treatment resistance to cytotoxic T lymphocyte–associated protein 4 (CTLA-4) and PD-L1 (programmed death-ligand 1) blockade.[39,40] In contrast, oral administration of *Bifidobacterium* potentiated the effect of PD-L1 therapy.[39] In humans, a study of a cohort of patients with renal cell carcinoma, urothelial carcinoma, and advanced non--small cell lung cancer found that patients treated with antibiotics before or shortly after the administration of immune checkpoint blockade had significantly shorter PFS and overall survival.[41] Moreover, *Akkermansia muciniphila* was found to be the critical organism, whereby oral supplementation of the bacteria to antibiotic-treated mice restored responsiveness to immunotherapy.[41]

In light of the newly discovered relationship between the microbiome and anticancer therapy responsiveness, it is conceivable that response to BCG can also be influenced by interactions with the commensal bacteria in the genitourinary tract. There is already evidence that bacillus binding, thought to be mediated by interactions between the bacterial cell wall and fibronectin in the urothelium,[42] can be affected by the presence of *Lactobacillus iners*.[43] Whether the intravesical microbiome can influence the outcomes of BCG therapy in other ways remains to be seen.

MECHANISTIC FACTORS

Despite decades of research, many questions regarding BCG's mechanism of action remain unanswered. A strategy to understand its mechanism has been to compare the immune response engendered in responders versus nonresponders and attempt to gain insight from the differences seen. Early efforts attempted to correlate differences in clinical immune response before and after BCG with therapeutic efficacy. Because skin reactivity to purified protein derivative (PPD) is the gold standard to detect antituberculin immunity, some investigators postulated that it can be used to characterize pretreatment BCG-specific immunity and predict improved antitumor response. Although earlier studies did not find a clear correlation,[44,45] 1 recent study by Biot and colleagues[46] found RFS to be significantly improved in patients with positive PPD. Results from this study have prompted the launch of SWOG 1602, a randomized phase III clinical trial examining the effect of priming and boost response to BCG.[47]

In addition, side effects of BCG treatment have also been used to predict response. It has been reported that patients who developed fevers during treatment have significantly lower recurrence rates.[45] Subsequently, an analysis of the EORTC 30911 results also indicated improved response rates in patients with significant side effects.[48] However, this observation could also be caused by the responders continuing to receive longer treatment courses of BCG, and thus reporting additional side effects. When limited to patients with and without symptoms within 6 months of treatment, no difference was found in RFS.

Investigating further, many studies have interrogated the difference between the cellular and cytokine response after BCG treatment. Higher levels of leukocyturia following BCG induction were associated with improved response.[49] Specifically, polymorphonuclear cells, through the production of TRAIL, were implicated as the effector cells of cytotoxicity.[50]

In addition, molecules associated with antigen presentation, such as heat shock protein (HSP) 90, are thought to play an integral part in facilitating effector cell recruitment and are necessary for treatment success.[51] A greater increase in major histocompatibility complex (MHC) class I expression, especially on the tumor cells, has also been found to predict higher RFS after treatment.[52,53] Intriguingly, MHC II and intercellular adhesion molecule 1 (ICAM1), which are typically restricted to immune cells, have also been found on cancer cells in BCG responders.[54,55] Note that the expression of these molecules is thought to be influenced by interferon, which is upregulated during BCG treatment.

Besides tumor cells, antigen-presenting cells (APCs) may also contribute to the recruitment and activation of effector cells on exposure to BCG.[56] However, whether the presence of APCs portends treatment success is unclear. Although immature dendritic cells (DCs) have been detected more frequently in the urine of BCG responders,[57] high levels of mature, tumor-infiltrating DCs have also been shown to predict treatment failure.[58] Similarly, antagonistic effects from different subsets of macrophages may differentially tip the balance toward treatment success or failure. Although those participating in T-helper 1 (Th1) response lead to tumor cell killing (M1), others involved in Th2 response are thought to stimulate cancer growth (M2). Along these lines, tumor-infiltrating cluster of differentiation (CD) 68+ tumor-associated macrophages were found to predict higher recurrence rates after BCG, indicating their involvement in the inflammatory circuit promoting tumor progression.[58,59]

In addition, it is unknown which cells are the key effectors in the BCG-elicited antitumor immune response. Early studies indicated that BCG-induced activity was lost in mice lacking lymphocytes, suggesting that these cells are necessary for the antitumor response.[60] This theory was supported by IHC studies showing increased numbers of CD4+ T cells after BCG treatment.[55,61] Moreover, the number of CD4+ T cells and CD4/CD8 ratio in the pretreated tumors were found to be predictive of treatment response.[62] In other studies, natural killer (NK) cells were found to be crucial for BCG-induced cytotoxicity.[63] In a small study, NK cell and tumor interactions were found to be stronger in BCG responders than in non-responders.[64] Without knowledge of the putative cytotoxic agent, it is difficult to pinpoint the cytotoxic response leading to treatment success.

Despite this lack of knowledge, insights can be obtained from the posttreatment immunogenic response. To this end, cytokine and chemokine profiles engendered after BCG instillation have been correlated with treatment success. Generation of the aforementioned Th1 polarized immune response is essential for an effective antitumor treatment. It is hypothesized that BCG is effective only when the tumor microenvironment (TME) converts from Th2 to Th1, and has no effect on the microenvironments already polarized to Th1.[65] Quantification of eosinophil infiltration and degranulation (Th2 polarized) and the ratio of GATA-3+ (high in Th2-polarized TME) to T-bet+ lymphocytes (high in Th1-polarized TME) predicted BCG failure.[65] The predictive value of GATA-3+/T-bet+ ratio has subsequently been validated.[66]

Urinary cytokines levels may also be used to predict treatment success. IL-2, a canonical Th1 cytokine secreted by CD4+ T cells thought to stimulate proliferation and maturation of several downstream effectors, is detected in larger quantities in the urine collected from BCG responder than from non-responders.[67] Furthermore, IL-2 levels peak earlier than IL-10 levels (surrogate for Th2 response) in responders, pushing the TME toward a Th1 response.[68,69] High IL-10 levels indicating a robust Th2 response, did not preclude treatment success.[31,68,69] Other investigators found that it was the relative levels of the counteracting cytokines, rather than their absolute values, that predicted treatment outcomes. For instance, the ratio between IL-6 and IL-10 had 83% sensitivity and 76% specificity in predicting recurrence after BCG.[70,71]

Several other cytokines have been identified to be differentially expressed in the urine of responders and non-responders. Higher levels of IL-8 after BCG therapy significantly correlated with longer CSS.[72] Other cytokines identified to be potential predictors of response include IL-18,[72] TNF-α,[73] IL-12,[66] and TRAIL.[50] The fact that a multitude of cytokines are related to treatment success is reflective of the complexity of the immune response resulting from BCG instillation. The authors prospectively tested the hypothesis that a panel of urinary cytokines can accurately assess the multifaceted immune response generated by intravesical BCG.[74] In a prospective study of 125 patients, urine was collected at various time points and multiple cytokines assessed. Various time point and ratio combinations were studied using computational analysis. After extensive modeling, the inducible levels of cytokines at the last (sixth) BCG instillation, calculated as the difference between preinstillation levels and postinstillation levels (4 hours after BCG), was most predictive of response. The number of cytokines required was then reduced to the minimum required to retain predictive power. A nomogram (CyPRIT [cytokine panel for response to intravesical therapy]) using a panel of 9 cytokines (IL-2, IL-6, IL-8, IL-18, IL-1ra, TRAIL, IFN-g, IL-12[p70], and TNF-α) had an accuracy of 85.5% in predicting response to BCG (95% confidence interval, 77.9%–93.1%) (Fig. 1). Efforts to validate the use of CyPRIT are currently underway.

Results from these studies not only shed light on how to predict treatment success but also helped to construct a basic framework underpinning BCG-induced antitumor immunity (Fig. 2): after attachment and uptake, BCG induces an innate immune response, attracting immune cell infiltrate, leading to the development of a Th1-polarized adaptive immune response.[75] Nonetheless, the question remains whether the antitumor response is directed specifically toward the tumor cells or merely a byproduct of BCG-specific immunity.[75] Furthermore, which are the key effector cells carrying out the cytotoxic activity? What is the cytokine profile required within the TME to foster such cytotoxicity? Until these questions are answered, it will be difficult to accurately predict response to BCG.

FUTURE DIRECTIONS

To answer these questions, some clues can be gleaned from immunotherapy research in other cancer systems. Much has been learned over the years about the criteria for generating an effective antineoplastic immune response. Chen and Mellman[76] summarized the key steps in the cancer-immunity cycle (Fig. 3), whereby neoantigens from the cancer cells are released and captured by DCs for processing; DCs subsequently present the captured antigens on MHC I and MHC II molecules to T cells, resulting in their priming and activation; activated effector T cells then travel to and infiltrate the tumor bed, recognizing neoantigens expressed by cancer cells; the cancer cells are recognized via the interaction between the T-cell receptor and its cognate antigen bound to MHC I and is killed

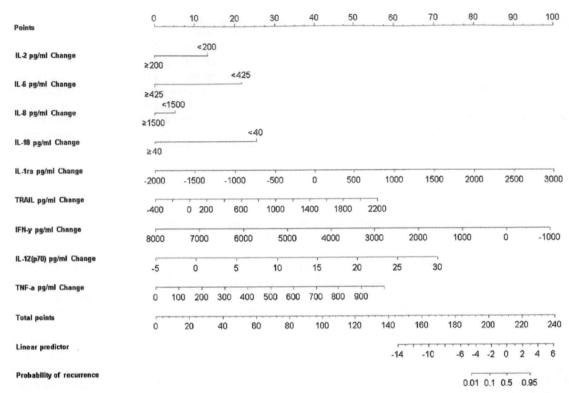

Fig. 1. CyPRIT nomogram for calculating the risk of recurrence using changes in urinary cytokine levels from immediately before to 4 hours after instillation of BCG at the last dose of induction (ie, at 6 weeks). (*From* Kamat AM, Briggman J, Urbauer DL, Svatek R, Nogueras Gonzalez GM, Anderson R, et al. Cytokine Panel for Response to Intravesical Therapy (CyPRIT): Nomogram of Changes in Urinary Cytokine Levels Predicts Patient Response to Bacillus Calmette-Guerin. Eur Urol. 2016;69(2):197-200; with permission.)

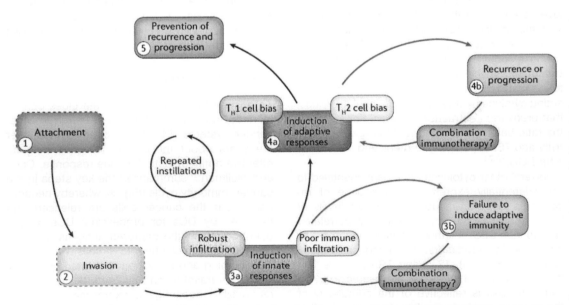

Fig. 2. Basic framework of the mechanism of BCG-induced antitumor immunity. (*From* Pettenati C, Ingersoll MA. Mechanisms of BCG immunotherapy and its outlook for bladder cancer. Nature Reviews Urology. 2018:1; with permission.)

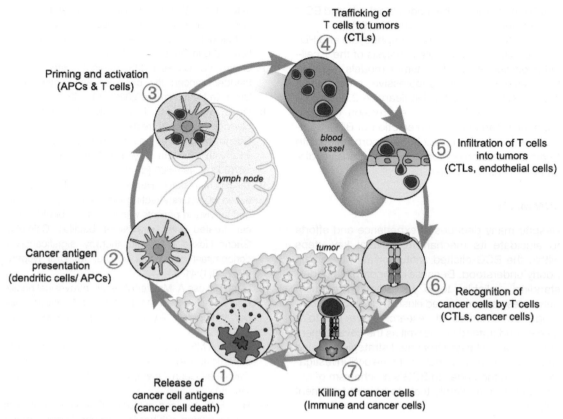

Fig. 3. The cancer-immunity cycle. CTLs, cytotoxic T lymphocytes. (*From* Chen DS, Mellman I. Oncology meets immunology: the cancer-immunity cycle. Immunity. 2013;39(1):1-10; with permission.)

by the effector T cell.[76] Within this system, BCG presumably facilitates the release of neoantigens and their presentation on DCs.

Because the BCG-mediated innate immune response is thought to be critical for downstream antitumor toxicity, methods to measure its activation may predict treatment efficacy. In melanoma, type I IFN production by the activated DCs is necessary for CD8+ effector T-cell priming against tumor antigens to give rise to the T cell–infiltrated TME.[77] In turn, through experiments using a series of knockout mice, Woo and colleagues[78] confirmed that the stimulator of interferon genes (STING) pathway was critical for spontaneous T-cell priming against tumor antigens, and subsequent rejection of immunogenic tumors. STING is an adapter molecule that is activated by cytosolic DNA.[79,80] This pathway has been implicated in the activation of the innate immune system against DNA viruses and select autoimmune diseases.[81] The important role played by STING in the antitumor immunity has since been recapitulated in several other tumor models.[82,83]

In bladder cancer, IFN-α–based therapy has recently been shown to have antitumor activity In the BCG-unresponsive setting.[84] Whether STING activation plays a role in BCG-mediated response is unknown. Future studies interrogating STING activity in BCG responders and non-responders are awaited to elucidate its role in BCG-mediated cytotoxicity.

Furthermore, treatment failure to immunotherapy has been observed even in patients with robust T-cell infiltrates directed against tumor antigens. Ex vivo analysis of these tumor antigen–specific T cells reveals various degrees of dysfunction.[85] This finding suggests that tumor progression, despite the adequately mounted adaptive immunity, can be caused by immunosuppressive mechanisms acting at the level of the TME. In support of this hypothesis, higher recurrence rates were found in patients with CD25hi or FOXP3+ T lymphocytes in pretreatment tumor samples.[62] In addition, high expression of PD-L1 in BCG granulomata was predictive of BCG failure.[86] Armed with several new agents approved in the metastatic MIBC setting,[87] clinical trials combining immune checkpoint blockade and BCG are currently underway (NCT02792192).

In addition to regulatory T lymphocytes and PD-L1 overexpression, detailed analysis of the T cell–inflamed subset of other tumor models revealed that several immune-suppressive mechanisms are present, including indoleamine-2,3-dioxygenase (IDO).[88] Whether the expression of these molecules can aid in the prediction of BCG treatment efficacy and possibly be incorporated into treatment strategies for BCG-unresponsive disease remains to be seen.

SUMMARY

Despite many decades of experience and efforts to elucidate its mechanism, several key steps within the BCG-elicited antitumor activity remain poorly understood. Because of incomplete understanding, reliable tools to predict treatment outcomes have remained elusive. However, promising new avenues of research have led to a deeper understanding, as well as the development of new diagnostic and treatment strategies. Armed with these, it is only a matter of time until investigators "crack the code" to BCG's mechanism of action and design reliable tools to predict treatment response.

REFERENCES

1. Morales A, Eidinger D, Bruce AW. Intracavitary Bacillus Calmette-Guerin in the treatment of superficial bladder tumors. J Urol 1976;116(2):180–3.
2. Cambier S, Sylvester RJ, Collette L, et al. EORTC nomograms and risk groups for predicting recurrence, progression, and disease-specific and overall survival in non-muscle-invasive stage Ta-T1 urothelial bladder cancer patients treated with 1-3 years of maintenance Bacillus Calmette-Guerin. Eur Urol 2016;69(1):60–9.
3. Fernandez-Gomez J, Solsona E, Unda M, et al. Prognostic factors in patients with non-muscle-invasive bladder cancer treated with bacillus Calmette-Guerin: multivariate analysis of data from four randomized CUETO trials. Eur Urol 2008; 53(5):992–1001.
4. van den Bosch S, Alfred Witjes J. Long-term cancer-specific survival in patients with high-risk, non-muscle-invasive bladder cancer and tumour progression: a systematic review. Eur Urol 2011;60(3): 493–500.
5. Fernandez-Gomez J, Madero R, Solsona E, et al. Predicting nonmuscle invasive bladder cancer recurrence and progression in patients treated with bacillus Calmette-Guerin: the CUETO scoring model. J Urol 2009;182(5):2195–203.
6. Martin-Doyle W, Leow JJ, Orsola A, et al. Improving selection criteria for early cystectomy in high-grade t1 bladder cancer: a meta-analysis of 15,215 patients. J Clin Oncol 2015;33(6):643–50.
7. Chang SS, Cookson MS. Radical cystectomy for bladder cancer: the case for early intervention. Urol Clin North Am 2005;32(2):147–55.
8. Davis JW, Sheth SI, Doviak MJ, et al. Superficial bladder carcinoma treated with bacillus Calmette-Guerin: progression-free and disease specific survival with minimum 10-year followup. J Urol 2002; 167(2 Pt 1):494–500 [discussion: 501].
9. Takashi M, Wakai K, Hattori T, et al. Multivariate evaluation of factors affecting recurrence, progression, and survival in patients with superficial bladder cancer treated with intravesical bacillus Calmette-Guerin (Tokyo 172 strain) therapy: significance of concomitant carcinoma in situ. Int Urol Nephrol 2002;33(1):41–7.
10. Hurle R, Losa A, Manzetti A, et al. Intravesical bacille Calmette-Guerin in Stage T1 grade 3 bladder cancer therapy: a 7-year follow-up. Urology 1999; 54(2):258–63.
11. Cookson MS, Sarosdy MF. Management of stage T1 superficial bladder cancer with intravesical bacillus Calmette-Guerin therapy. J Urol 1992;148(3): 797–801.
12. Herr HW. Age and outcome of superficial bladder cancer treated with bacille Calmette-Guerin therapy. Urology 2007;70(1):65–8.
13. Hurle R, Losa A, Ranieri A, et al. Low dose Pasteur bacillus Calmette-Guerin regimen in stage T1, grade 3 bladder cancer therapy. J Urol 1996;156(5):1602–5.
14. Pansadoro V, Emiliozzi P, de Paula F, et al. Long-term follow-up of G3T1 transitional cell carcinoma of the bladder treated with intravesical bacille Calmette-Guerin: 18-year experience. Urology 2002;59(2):227–31.
15. Kamat AM, Li R, O'Donnell MA, et al. Predicting response to intravesical bacillus Calmette-guerin immunotherapy: are we there yet? a systematic review. Eur Urol 2018;73(5):738–48.
16. Lacombe L, Dalbagni G, Zhang ZF, et al. Overexpression of p53 protein in a high-risk population of patients with superficial bladder cancer before and after bacillus Calmette-Guerin therapy: correlation to clinical outcome. J Clin Oncol 1996;14(10): 2646–52.
17. Pages F, Flam TA, Vieillefond A, et al. p53 status does not predict initial clinical response to bacillus Calmette-Guerin intravesical therapy in T1 bladder tumors. J Urol 1998;159(3):1079–84.
18. Ovesen H, Horn T, Steven K. Long-term efficacy of intravesical bacillus Calmette-Guerin for carcinoma in situ: relationship of progression to histological response and p53 nuclear accumulation. J Urol 1997;157(5):1655–9.

19. Schmitz-Drager BJ, Goebell PJ, Ebert T, et al. p53 immunohistochemistry as a prognostic marker in bladder cancer. Playground for urology scientists? Eur Urol 2000;38(6):691–9 [discussion: 700].

20. Halling KC, King W, Sokolova IA, et al. A comparison of cytology and fluorescence in situ hybridization for the detection of urothelial carcinoma. J Urol 2000; 164(5):1768–75.

21. Kamat AM, Dickstein RJ, Messetti F, et al. Use of fluorescence in situ hybridization to predict response to bacillus Calmette-Guerin therapy for bladder cancer: results of a prospective trial. J Urol 2012;187(3):862–7.

22. Kamat AM, Willis DL, Dickstein RJ, et al. Novel fluorescence in situ hybridization-based definition of bacille Calmette-Guerin (BCG) failure for use in enhancing recruitment into clinical trials of intravesical therapies. BJU Int 2016;117(5):754–60.

23. Faltas BM, Prandi D, Tagawa ST, et al. Clonal evolution of chemotherapy-resistant urothelial carcinoma. Nat Genet 2016;48(12):1490–9.

24. Van Allen EM, Mouw KW, Kim P, et al. Somatic ERCC2 mutations correlate with cisplatin sensitivity in muscle-invasive urothelial carcinoma. Cancer Discov 2014;4(10):1140–53.

25. Seiler R, Ashab HA, Erho N, et al. Impact of molecular Subtypes in muscle-invasive bladder cancer on predicting response and survival after neoadjuvant chemotherapy. Eur Urol 2017;72(4):544–54.

26. Gu J, Zhao H, Dinney CP, et al. Nucleotide excision repair gene polymorphisms and recurrence after treatment for superficial bladder cancer. Clin Cancer Res 2005;11(4):1408–15.

27. Meeks JJ, Carneiro BA, Pai SG, et al. Genomic characterization of high-risk non-muscle invasive bladder cancer. Oncotarget 2016;7(46):75176–84.

28. Hedegaard J, Lamy P, Nordentoft I, et al. Comprehensive transcriptional analysis of early-stage urothelial carcinoma. Cancer Cell 2016;30(1):27–42.

29. Pietzak EJ, Bagrodia A, Cha EK, et al. Next-generation sequencing of nonmuscle invasive bladder cancer reveals potential biomarkers and rational therapeutic targets. Eur Urol 2017;72(6):952–9.

30. Palou J, Sylvester RJ, Faba OR, et al. Female gender and carcinoma in situ in the prostatic urethra are prognostic factors for recurrence, progression, and disease-specific mortality in T1G3 bladder cancer patients treated with bacillus Calmette-Guerin. Eur Urol 2012;62(1):118–25.

31. Saint F, Patard JJ, Maille P, et al. Prognostic value of a T helper 1 urinary cytokine response after intravesical bacillus Calmette-Guerin treatment for superficial bladder cancer. J Urol 2002;167(1):364–7.

32. Morales EE, Grill S, Svatek RS, et al. Finasteride reduces risk of bladder cancer in a large prospective screening study. Eur Urol 2016;69(3): 407–10.

33. Joudi FN, Smith BJ, O'Donnell MA, et al. The impact of age on the response of patients with superficial bladder cancer to intravesical immunotherapy. J Urol 2006;175(5):1634–9 [discussion: 1639–40].

34. Oddens JR, Sylvester RJ, Brausi MA, et al. The effect of age on the efficacy of maintenance bacillus Calmette-Guerin relative to maintenance epirubicin in patients with stage Ta T1 urothelial bladder cancer: results from EORTC genito-urinary group study 30911. Eur Urol 2014;66(4):694–701.

35. Leibovici D, Grossman HB, Dinney CP, et al. Polymorphisms in inflammation genes and bladder cancer: from initiation to recurrence, progression, and survival. J Clin Oncol 2005;23(24):5746–56.

36. Lima L, Oliveira D, Ferreira JA, et al. The role of functional polymorphisms in immune response genes as biomarkers of bacille Calmette-Guerin (BCG) immunotherapy outcome in bladder cancer: establishment of a predictive profile in a Southern Europe population. BJU Int 2015;116(5):753–63.

37. Spanogiannopoulos P, Bess EN, Carmody RN, et al. The microbial pharmacists within us: a metagenomic view of xenobiotic metabolism. Nat Rev Microbiol 2016;14(5):273.

38. Geller LT, Barzily-Rokni M, Danino T, et al. Potential role of intratumor bacteria in mediating tumor resistance to the chemotherapeutic drug gemcitabine. Science 2017;357(6356):1156–60.

39. Sivan A, Corrales L, Hubert N, et al. Commensal Bifidobacterium promotes antitumor immunity and facilitates anti–PD-L1 efficacy. Science 2015; 350(6264):1084–9.

40. Vétizou M, Pitt JM, Daillère R, et al. Anticancer immunotherapy by CTLA-4 blockade relies on the gut microbiota. Science 2015;350(6264):1079–84.

41. Routy B, Le Chatelier E, Derosa L, et al. Gut microbiome influences efficacy of PD-1–based immunotherapy against epithelial tumors. Science 2018; 359(6371):91–7.

42. Bevers R, Kurth K, Schamhart D. Role of urothelial cells in BCG immunotherapy for superficial bladder cancer. Br J Cancer 2004;91(4):607.

43. McMillan A, Macklaim JM, Burton JP, et al. Adhesion of Lactobacillus iners AB-1 to human fibronectin: a key mediator for persistence in the vagina? Reprod Sci 2013;20(7):791–6.

44. Bilen CY, Inci K, Erkan I, et al. The predictive value of purified protein derivative results on complications and prognosis in patients with bladder cancer treated with bacillus Calmette-Guerin. J Urol 2003; 169(5):1702–5.

45. Luftenegger W, Ackermann DK, Futterlieb A, et al. Intravesical versus intravesical plus intradermal bacillus Calmette-Guerin: a prospective randomized study in patients with recurrent superficial bladder tumors. J Urol 1996;155(2):483–7.

46. Biot C, Rentsch CA, Gsponer JR, et al. Preexisting BCG-specific T cells improve intravesical immunotherapy for bladder cancer. Sci Transl Med 2012; 4(137):137ra72.

47. Svatek RS, Tangen C, Delacroix S, et al. Background and update for S1602 "a phase III randomized trial to evaluate the influence of BCG strain differences and T cell priming with intradermal BCG before intravesical therapy for BCG-naive high-grade non-muscle-invasive bladder cancer. Eur Urol Focus 2018;4(4):522–4.

48. Sylvester RJ, van der Meijden AP, Oosterlinck W, et al. The side effects of Bacillus Calmette-Guerin in the treatment of Ta T1 bladder cancer do not predict its efficacy: results from a European Organisation for Research and Treatment of Cancer Genito-Urinary Group Phase III Trial. Eur Urol 2003;44(4): 423–8.

49. Saint F, Patard JJ, Irani J, et al. Leukocyturia as a predictor of tolerance and efficacy of intravesical BCG maintenance therapy for superficial bladder cancer. Urology 2001;57(4):617–21 [discussion: 621–2].

50. Ludwig AT, Moore JM, Luo Y, et al. Tumor necrosis factor-related apoptosis-inducing ligand: a novel mechanism for Bacillus Calmette-Guerin-induced antitumor activity. Cancer Res 2004;64(10):3386–90.

51. Lebret T, Watson RW, Molinie V, et al. HSP90 expression: a new predictive factor for BCG response in stage Ta-T1 grade 3 bladder tumours. Eur Urol 2007;51(1):161–6 [discussion: 106–7].

52. Videira PA, Calais FM, Correia M, et al. Efficacy of bacille Calmette-Guerin immunotherapy predicted by expression of antigen-presenting molecules and chemokines. Urology 2009;74(4):944–50.

53. Kitamura H, Torigoe T, Honma I, et al. Effect of human leukocyte antigen class I expression of tumor cells on outcome of intravesical instillation of bacillus calmette-guerin immunotherapy for bladder cancer. Clin Cancer Res 2006;12(15):4641–4.

54. Jackson AM, Alexandroff AB, McIntyre M, et al. Induction of ICAM 1 expression on bladder tumours by BCG immunotherapy. J Clin Pathol 1994;47(4): 309–12.

55. Prescott S, James K, Hargreave TB, et al. Intravesical Evans strain BCG therapy: quantitative immunohistochemical analysis of the immune response within the bladder wall. J Urol 1992;147(6):1636–42.

56. Naoe M, Ogawa Y, Takeshita K, et al. Bacillus Calmette-Guerin-pulsed dendritic cells stimulate natural killer T cells and gammadeltaT cells. Int J Urol 2007;14(6):532–8 [discussion: 508].

57. Beatty JD, Islam S, North ME, et al. Urine dendritic cells: a noninvasive probe for immune activity in bladder cancer? BJU Int 2004;94(9):1377–83.

58. Ayari C, LaRue H, Hovington H, et al. Bladder tumor infiltrating mature dendritic cells and macrophages as predictors of response to bacillus Calmette-Guerin immunotherapy. Eur Urol 2009;55(6): 1386–95.

59. Takayama H, Nishimura K, Tsujimura A, et al. Increased infiltration of tumor associated macrophages is associated with poor prognosis of bladder carcinoma in situ after intravesical bacillus Calmette-Guerin instillation. J Urol 2009;181(4): 1894–900.

60. Ratliff TL, Palmer JO, McGarr JA, et al. Intravesical Bacillus Calmette-Guerin therapy for murine bladder tumors: initiation of the response by fibronectin-mediated attachment of Bacillus Calmette-Guerin. Cancer Res 1987;47(7):1762–6.

61. Bohle A, Gerdes J, Ulmer AJ, et al. Effects of local bacillus Calmette-Guerin therapy in patients with bladder carcinoma on immunocompetent cells of the bladder wall. J Urol 1990;144(1):53–8.

62. Pichler R, Fritz J, Zavadil C, et al. Tumor-infiltrating immune cell subpopulations influence the oncologic outcome after intravesical bacillus calmette-guerin therapy in bladder cancer. Oncotarget 2016;7(26): 39916–30.

63. Brandau S, Riemensberger J, Jacobsen M, et al. NK cells are essential for effective BCG immunotherapy. Int J Cancer 2001;92(5):697–702.

64. Yutkin V, Pode D, Pikarsky E, et al. The expression level of ligands for natural killer cell receptors predicts response to bacillus Calmette-Guerin therapy: a pilot study. J Urol 2007;178(6):2660–4.

65. Nunez-Nateras R, Castle EP, Protheroe CA, et al. Predicting response to bacillus Calmette-Guerin (BCG) in patients with carcinoma in situ of the bladder. Urol Oncol 2014;32(1):45.e23-30.

66. Pichler R, Gruenbacher G, Culig Z, et al. Intratumoral Th2 predisposition combines with an increased Th1 functional phenotype in clinical response to intravesical BCG in bladder cancer. Cancer Immunol Immunother 2017;66(4):427–40.

67. Saint F, Kurth N, Maille P, et al. Urinary IL-2 assay for monitoring intravesical bacillus Calmette-Guerin response of superficial bladder cancer during induction course and maintenance therapy. Int J Cancer 2003;107(3):434–40.

68. Saint F, Salomon L, Quintela R, et al. Do prognostic parameters of remission versus relapse after Bacillus Calmette-Guerin (BCG) immunotherapy exist?. analysis of a quarter century of literature. Eur Urol 2003;43(4):351–60 [discussion: 360–1].

69. Nadler R, Luo Y, Zhao W, et al. Interleukin 10 induced augmentation of delayed-type hypersensitivity (DTH) enhances Mycobacterium bovis bacillus Calmette-Guerin (BCG) mediated antitumour activity. Clin Exp Immunol 2003;131(2): 206–16.

70. Cai T, Mazzoli S, Meacci F, et al. Interleukin-6/10 ratio as a prognostic marker of recurrence in patients

with intermediate risk urothelial bladder carcinoma. J Urol 2007;178(5):1906–11 [discussion: 1911–2].

71. Cai T, Nesi G, Mazzoli S, et al. Prediction of response to bacillus Calmette-Guerin treatment in non-muscle invasive bladder cancer patients through interleukin-6 and interleukin-10 ratio. Exp Ther Med 2012;4(3):459–64.

72. Thalmann GN, Sermier A, Rentsch C, et al. Urinary Interleukin-8 and 18 predict the response of superficial bladder cancer to intravesical therapy with bacillus Calmette-Guerin. J Urol 2000;164(6):2129–33.

73. Shintani Y, Sawada Y, Inagaki T, et al. Intravesical instillation therapy with bacillus Calmette-Guerin for superficial bladder cancer: study of the mechanism of bacillus Calmette-Guerin immunotherapy. Int J Urol 2007;14(2):140–6.

74. Kamat AM, Briggman J, Urbauer DL, et al. Cytokine panel for response to intravesical therapy (CyPRIT): nomogram of changes in urinary cytokine levels predicts patient response to bacillus Calmette-Guerin. Eur Urol 2016;69(2):197–200.

75. Pettenati C, Ingersoll MA. Mechanisms of BCG immunotherapy and its outlook for bladder cancer. Nat Rev Urol 2018;15(10):615–25.

76. Chen DS, Mellman I. Oncology meets immunology: the cancer-immunity cycle. Immunity 2013;39(1):1–10.

77. Fuertes MB, Woo S-R, Burnett B, et al. Type I interferon response and innate immune sensing of cancer. Trends Immunol 2013;34(2):67–73.

78. Woo S-R, Fuertes MB, Corrales L, et al. STING-dependent cytosolic DNA sensing mediates innate immune recognition of immunogenic tumors. Immunity 2014;41(5):830–42.

79. Ishikawa H, Barber GN. STING is an endoplasmic reticulum adaptor that facilitates innate immune signalling. Nature 2008;455(7213):674.

80. Sun L, Wu J, Du F, et al. Cyclic GMP-AMP synthase is a cytosolic DNA sensor that activates the type I interferon pathway. Science 2013;339(6121):786–91.

81. Ahn J, Gutman D, Saijo S, et al. STING manifests self DNA-dependent inflammatory disease. Proc Natl Acad Sci U S A 2012;109(47):19386–91.

82. Ohkuri T, Ghosh A, Kosaka A, et al. STING contributes to anti-glioma immunity via triggering type-I IFN signals in the tumor microenvironment. J Immunother Cancer 2014;2(3):P228.

83. Zhu Q, Man SM, Gurung P, et al. Cutting edge: STING mediates protection against colorectal tumorigenesis by governing the magnitude of intestinal inflammation. J Immunol 2014;193(10):4779–82.

84. Shore ND, Boorjian SA, Canter DJ, et al. Intravesical rAd-IFNalpha/Syn3 for patients with high-grade, bacillus Calmette-Guerin-refractory or relapsed non-muscle-invasive bladder cancer: a phase II randomized study. J Clin Oncol 2017;35(30):3410–6.

85. Harlin H, Meng Y, Peterson AC, et al. Chemokine expression in melanoma metastases associated with CD8+ T-cell recruitment. Cancer Res 2009;69(7):3077–85.

86. Inman BA, Sebo TJ, Frigola X, et al. PD-L1 (B7-H1) expression by urothelial carcinoma of the bladder and BCG-induced granulomata: associations with localized stage progression. Cancer 2007;109(8):1499–505.

87. Balar AV, Galsky MD, Rosenberg JE, et al. Atezolizumab as first-line treatment in cisplatin-ineligible patients with locally advanced and metastatic urothelial carcinoma: a single-arm, multicentre, phase 2 trial. Lancet 2017;389(10064):67–76.

88. Spranger S, Spaapen RM, Zha Y, et al. Up-regulation of PD-L1, IDO, and Tregs in the melanoma tumor microenvironment is driven by CD8+ T cells. Sci Transl Med 2013;5(200):200ra116.

Genomic and Therapeutic Landscape of Non-muscle-invasive Bladder Cancer

Lauren Folgosa Cooley, MD, PhD[a], Kimberly A. McLaughlin, BS, MS[a,b,c], Joshua J. Meeks, MD, PhD[a,b,c],*

KEYWORDS

- Bladder cancer • Mutation • Genomics • Immunotherapy • BCG

KEY POINTS

- Non–muscle-invasive bladder cancers (NMIBCs) are heterogeneous across stage and grades. The current treatment relies on clinical and pathologic parameters.
- Much less is known about the genetic features of NMIBC compared with muscle-invasive bladder cancer, and these discoveries may help identify targeted therapies.
- Ongoing investigations into immunotherapies for NMIBC are critical given shortages and differential responsiveness to bacillus Calmette-Guérin.

INTRODUCTION

Urothelial carcinoma (UC) is the fifth most common cancer in the United States. Of diagnosed patients, nearly 80% present with non–muscle-invasive bladder cancer (NMIBC), comprising tumor stages Ta, T1, and carcinoma in situ (CIS).[1] Each stage of NMIBC has recently been found to have distinct biological and molecular features, which may translate into clinical heterogeneity affecting recurrence, progression, and response to therapy.[2] Stage Ta tumors include papillary urothelial neoplasms of low malignant potential and low-grade and high-grade noninvasive papillary UC, which are predominated by luminal differentiation. Few Ta tumors progress to muscle-invasive

disease, but recurrence rates are high, requiring frequent intravesical therapy.[2] Alternatively, invasive cancers (stage T1) and preinvasive CIS are more likely to progress to muscle invasion and metastasis. Although most T1 tumors are high grade, all CIS is considered high grade and usually responsive or partially responsive to bacillus Calmette-Guérin (BCG) immunotherapy.[2]

The current treatment of NMIBC relies on clinical and pathologic parameters largely based on stage and grade, lacking individualization to tumor and host biology. However, recent advances in genomics technology pioneered by The Cancer Genome Atlas (TCGA) have facilitated the comprehensive analysis of genomic, epigenetic, and transcriptomic alterations across tumor types.[3,4]

Disclosure: L.F. Cooley and K.A. McLaughlin have nothing to disclose. J.J. Meeks is a consultant for Ferring and Astra Zeneca, receives honoraria from Janssen and Cold Genesys, and receives research funding from Epizyme, Abbvie, and Tesaro, with clinical trial support from Merck.

Funding: J.J. Meeks is supported by Department of Veterans Affairs (BX003692) and Department of Defense (W81XWH-18-0257) and an award from the John P. Hanson Foundation for Cancer Research (Milwaukee, WI).

[a] Department of Urology, Feinberg School of Medicine, Northwestern University, 300 East Superior Street, Tarry 16-703, Chicago, IL 60611, USA; [b] Department of Biochemistry, Northwestern University, Feinberg School of Medicine, Polsky Urologic Cancer Institute, Chicago, IL 60611, USA; [c] Robert H. Lurie Comprehensive Cancer Center, Northwestern University, Chicago, IL 60611, USA

* Corresponding author. Department of Urology, Feinberg School of Medicine, Northwestern University, 300 East Superior Street, Tarry 16-703, Chicago, IL 60611.

E-mail address: joshua.meeks@northwestern.edu

Urol Clin N Am 47 (2020) 35–46
https://doi.org/10.1016/j.ucl.2019.09.006
0094-0143/20/Published by Elsevier Inc.

These advances, coupled with ongoing research into new chemotherapeutic strategies for NMIBC, are intended to individualize future cancer treatment. This article highlights key features of tumor and host biology that may be applied for the risk stratification and treatment of NMIBC in this new era of precision medicine.

GENOMIC LANDSCAPE OF NON–MUSCLE-INVASIVE BLADDER CANCER

The heterogeneity of NMIBCs is derived from mutations, mutation signatures, chromosomal loss, and disruption of molecular pathways. **Fig. 1**A and B compare the heterogeneity of stage Ta and T1, as well as differential gene expression profiles of tumors with recurrence compared with nonrecurrence.[5,6]

Apolipoprotein B Messenger RNA Editing Enzyme Catalytic Polypeptidelike–Mediated Mutagenesis and Intratumor Heterogeneity

DNA is constantly under the stress of mutation and repair. Within a tumor, patterns of mutations may develop, termed a signature of this mutagenesis. These mutation signatures vary by age, tumor type, and origin of cancer. In bladder cancer, the predominant mutation signature is apolipoprotein B messenger RNA editing enzyme catalytic polypeptidelike (APOBEC) mediated.[7] APOBEC are a family of cytosine deaminases, which under physiologic conditions perform C>U editing of single-stranded DNA.[3] During cytosine deamination,

APOBEC catalyzes a 5'-T-phosphate-C-3' (TpC) to T, G, or A, which, if unregulated, can lead to hypermutation.[3,7,8] Therefore, in bladder cancer APOBEC activity has been associated with a high tumor mutation burden (TMB).[2] TCGA 2014 and 2017 analyses of muscle-invasive bladder cancer (MIBC) specimens showed APOBEC mutation patterns in 93% and 67%, respectively.[3,4] An increase in TMB reflects genomic stress but may be a good prognostic biomarker because MIBCs with higher TMB were associated with improved survival. When low APOBEC MIBCs were evaluated, our group identified an enrichment of oncogenes RAS and FGFR3, suggesting that processes driving APOBEC-mediated mutagenesis were complimentary to oncogene-induced tumor growth.[9] However, in NMIBC the TMB is at least 3-fold lower compared with MIBC[2] and enrichment of APOBEC signatures increases with stage and grade.[2,10] In an analysis of 140 Ta tumors, high-grade (GS2) tumors were more likely to be APOBEC enriched with high rates of recurrence.[2] Similarly, a prospective European multi-center collaboration (FP7:UROMOL), showed an association between high-risk NMIBC and APOBEC mutagenesis. Therein, class 2 tumors, which showed worse progression and higher rates of concomitant CIS, had increased APOBEC mutation signatures ($P = 3.4 \times 10^{-8}$) and expression of APOBEC3A and 3B.[10] In addition, APOBEC expression may vary over the lifetime of a tumor, especially in tumors with progression.[11,12] In a small cohort of 29 patients with serial biopsies,

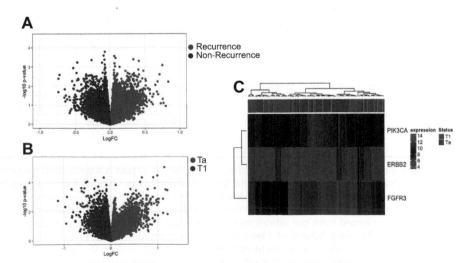

Fig. 1. Genomic characteristics of NMIBC. (A) Differential gene expression comparison between tumors that recur (red) and do not recur (blue) across all stages. (B) Differential comparison between Ta (red) and T1 (blue) tumors. (C) Lower-stage NMIBC (Ta, blue) is associated with increased fibroblast growth factor receptor 3 (FGFR3), stable ERBB2, and decreased cancer-associated phosphatidylinositol 3-kinase (PIK3CA) expression compared with T1 (red). Compared with FGFR3 levels, NMIBCs have variable expression of both ERBB2 and PIK3CA. NMIBC gene expression is from E-MTAB-1940 with visualization using GEO2R.[5,6]

Lamy and colleagues[11] found higher variance in TMB and increased APOBEC enrichment in patients who progressed (53%, 8 out of 15) compared with nonprogressors (7%, 1 out of 14) ($P<.009$). Whether tumors that progress have higher genomic instability with or from APOBEC-mediated repair is unknown.

Chromosomal Aberrations

Increase in copy number alterations and genomic instability is linked to higher stage and worse prognosis in bladder cancer. Furthermore, systematic loss of chromosome regions has been identified in patients with NMIBC, which have direct implications on prognosis.[2,13,14] Although most NMIBCs are diploid or near diploid, loss of specific regions is associated with higher recurrence.[2,15,16] A comparison of genetic aberrations in 28 Ta versus 28 T1 tumors found loss of 9q (54%), 9p (39%), Y (28%), and gain of 1q (14%) were more prevalent in Ta tumors, whereas loss of 2q (36%), 8p (32%), and 11p (21%) was more common in T1 tumors.[16] Hurst and colleagues[2] similarly reported loss of chromosome 9q in 41% of Ta tumors resulting in the supervised clustering of Ta tumors into GS1 (normal for 9q) or GS2 subtypes (loss of 9q). GS2 tumors were predominantly high grade ($P = .0053$), with 9q deletion present in 3.4% GS1 versus 87.3% GS2. Interestingly, loss of 9q has also been shown in normal urothelium adjacent to areas of tumor. This finding suggests loss of 9q may be an early marker of local genomic instability and may play a role early in the initiation of bladder cancer development.[2,17]

Candidate tumor suppressor genes on chromosome 9q that may play a role in bladder cancer pathogenesis are NOTCH1 and TSC1. NOTCH1, which acts predominantly as a tumor suppressor compared with family members NOTCH2 and 3, has been shown to be downregulated in bladder cancer, with inactivation of NOTCH1 occurring more frequently in high-grade tumors.[18–20] Rampias and colleagues[18] found Notch pathway or NOTCH1 mutation in 61% (44 out of 72) and 51% (37 out of 72) of bladder cancer specimens, respectively, with presence of mutation significantly correlating with risk of death ($P = .059$) and muscle-invasive disease ($P = .037$). Loss of TSC1, the negative regulator of mammalian target of rapamycin (mTOR), may be associated with increased cell growth and survival in NMIBC, and gene expression studies of GS2 tumors suggest increased activation of mTOR pathways in high-risk disease.[2] TSC1 would be an exciting target for NMIBC because everolimus may be a cost-effective therapy to prevent recurrence of GS2 tumors. Although everolimus has not been universally effective in metastatic urothelial cancer, unique responders with alterations in TSC1 and NF1 have been identified to have durable response.[21] Furthermore, a recent pilot study of rapamycin after cystectomy showed enhanced immune activity that may decrease tumor recurrence.[22]

RTK-RAS–Phosphatidylinositol 3-kinase Pathway (Fibroblast Growth Factor Receptor 3, ERBB2 (Erb-b2 Receptor Tyrosine Kinase 2), Cancer-Associated Phosphatidylinositol 3-kinase)

Fibroblast growth factor receptor 3

NMIBCs have features of differentiated urothelium with consistent activation of the fibroblast growth factor receptor 3 (FGFR3) and Ras pathways. FGFR3 signals through Ras (RAS-MAPK-ERK pathway) and regulates cell cycle entry and proliferation. Mutation in FGFR3 is most common in Ta tumors ($\sim$80%), with decreased frequency noted in high-grade Ta (59%), T1 (10%–34%), and MIBC (10%–20%) (**Fig. 1**C).[23–27] A pooled meta-analysis by Liu and colleagues[28] reiterated these findings, showing increased frequency of FGFR3 mutation in low-grade (Relative Risk (RR), 2.948; 95% confidence interval [CI], 2.357–3.688) and early-stage (RR = 2.845; 95% CI = 2.145–3.773) bladder cancer as well as an association with improved disease-free, progression-free, and recurrence-free survival. Of those NMIBCs that progress to MIBC, mutation of FGFR3 was found in 25% of tumors compared with only 7% of tumors that presented as MIBC.[27]

FGFR3 fusion proteins are also implicated in bladder cancer pathogenesis, with FGFR3-TACC3 fusions being the most common. TACC3 is upstream of FGFR3 signaling and this fusion protein causes constitutive activation of the MAPK-ERK pathway, unregulated cell proliferation, and promotion of aneuploidy.[7] Although more commonly associated with MIBC, FGFR3-TACC3 fusions have been identified in NMIBC cell lines and reported in 1 Ta tumor (1 out of 23, low-grade Ta) by Pietzak and colleagues.[4,27,29–31] Small molecule inhibitors targeting FGFR3 have been used in metastatic bladder cancer. Although dovitinib was considered to be unsuccessful for BCG-refractory bladder cancer, with a complete response rate of only 8%, targeting tumors with FGFR3 alterations has been associated with improved response.[31] In a phase II trial of erdafitinib for metastatic UC with FGFR3 alterations, the overall response rate was 40% and, of those treated with 8 mg, 76% had a reduction in size of their largest tumor. However, the median duration of response was only 5.6 months (4.2–7.2 months).[32] In a similar study of patients with metastatic UC with *FGFR3* alterations, a pan-FGFR–blocking antagonist, BGJ398, was administered in a 3-weeks-on, 1-week-off cycle. The overall response rate was 25.4%, with disease stabilization in 38.8% and response duration of 5.06 months (95% CI, 3.91–7.36 months).[33] Interestingly, *FGFR3* mutations were identified by cell-free DNA in 68% of patients, which could translate to methods of sampling tumor or urine without the need for recurrent biopsy.[33] In addition, there are 2 additional clinical trials assessing FGFR3 blockade in patients with metastatic UC harboring *FGFR3* mutations (NCT02365597, NCT02038673). Although most published results on *FGFR3* alterations are in metastatic disease, the high frequency of *FGFR3* mutation in NMIBC suggests that *FGFR3* may be a rational target in NMIBC as well depending on the tolerability of each therapy.

ERBB2

ERBB2 encodes human epidermal growth factor receptor 2 (Her2), which is mitogenic for cell growth and survival.[34] Of all cancer types, *ERBB2* amplification occurs third most commonly in bladder cancer and is associated with high-risk features including risk of progression and concomitant CIS in NMIBC specimens.[35–37] Pietzak and colleagues[27] characterized genomic alterations in 105 NMIBCs (12 high-grade Tis, 23 low-grade Ta, 12 high-grade Ta, and 28 high-grade T1) and found *ERBB2* mutations were only present in high-grade NMIBC tumors apart from a single low-grade Ta tumor. *ERBB2* mutations were associated with higher-stage (HGT1, ~25%; HGTa, ~20%; LGTa, ~5%; P = .05) and high-grade (HGTa, ~20% vs LGTa, ~5%%; P = .01) tumors compared with *FGFR3* mutations, which were present in only 39% of high-grade tumors and more characteristic of low-grade, low-stage NMIBC (LGTa, ~80%; HGTa, ~60%; HGT1 ~35%). In UROMOL, *ERBB2* mutations were more common in class 2 tumors and were altered in 20% of tumors.[10] These findings suggest *FGFR3* alterations may be more common in low-grade, noninvasive tumors, whereas *ERBB2* alteration is a driver of higher-stage and higher-grade tumors. The authors examined the expression across Ta and T1 (see **Fig. 1**C) and found little association with stage.

Cancer-associated phosphatidylinositol 3-kinase

The phosphatidylinositol 3-kinase (PI3K)/mTOR/protein kinase B (AKT) pathway may provide growth advantage during the initiation of cancer. *PIK3CA* (cancer-associated phosphatidylinositol 3-kinase) encodes the catalytic subunit of PI3K and is more frequently mutated in NMIBC compared with MIBC (Ta, 40%–50%[17]; T1, 6%–20%[17]; MIBC, 22%[4]).[4,17,38] Hurst and colleagues[2,17] found that 40% to 50% of Ta tumors and 6% to 20% of T1 tumors harbored a *PIK3CA* mutation, which typically occurred as a point mutation in a codon critical for catalytic activity. The UROMOL series identified mTOR/PI3K alterations in 59% of tumors with *NF1* mutations in 24%, *PIK3CA* in 23%, and *PIKR* in 9% of patients with mutations in *PIK3CA* commonly coexisting with *FGFR3* mutations.[2,10,38] Our evaluation of 25 T1 tumors did not find a significant difference in frequency of *PIK3CA* mutations in high-risk NMIBC specimens (T1 high grade or Ta high grade with CIS) from patients who progressed to muscle-invasive or metastatic stages compared with nonprogressors.[39] Collectively, this finding suggests this mutation may play a role early in bladder cancer initiation or recurrence rather than disease progression.

Chromatin-Modifying Genes (ARID1A, KDM6A) and Epigenetic Dysregulation

Chromatin-modifying genes (CMGs) are commonly mutated across cancer types and serve as regulators of gene expression.[4,29] Pietzak and colleagues[27] found that the 2 most commonly mutated CMGs in NMIBC were *KDM6A* (38%) and *ARID1A* (28%). Although neither mutation correlated statistically with tumor stage or grade, *KDM6A* mutation frequency decreased with increasing grade/stage (52% LGTa, 38% HGTa, 32% HGT1, 25% Memorial Sloan Kettering (MSK)-MIBC, 24% TCGA-MIBC), whereas *ARID1A* mutation frequency tended to increase with increasing grade/stage (9% LGTa, 28% HGTa, 18% HGT1, 30% MSK-MIBC, 24% TCGA-MIBC). An increased frequency of *KDM6A* mutations was found in female patients with Ta tumors (20 out of 27, 72%) compared with men (23 out of 55, 42%; P = .0092). KDM6A is not X inactivated in women and the increased frequency of mutations may suggest increased pressure on *KDM6A* in women with 2 expressed copies.[2] Tumors with mutations of *KDM6A* may have increased H3K27me3 from unbalanced epigenetic regulation at H3K27. To counter increased H3K27me3, treatment with an EZH2-inhibitor may normalize enhancer methylation.[40] Our research group has also found increased sensitivity to EZH2 inhibitors in tumors with *KMT2C* alteration that disrupts recruitment of KDM6A (under investigation).

ARID1A mutation has been associated with increasing stage (24% MIBC vs 20% NMIBC) and aggressiveness.[7,27] Pietzak and colleagues[27] reported that alterations in *ARID1A* were significantly associated with increased risk of recurrence, which may correspond with increased aggressiveness or BCG-resistance (hazard ratio [HR], 3.14; 95% CI, 1.51–6.51; *P* = .002). With further investigation, *ARID1A* may serve as a predictive biomarker in patients undergoing BCG therapy or a potential therapeutic target to enhance BCG response (discussed later).

Telomerase Reverse Transcriptase Promoter

Enzymatic activation of telomerase maintains the 3′ telomere length at the ends of chromosomes to avoid senescence and apoptosis and promote cellular lifespan. Promoter mutations in the telomerase reverse transcriptase gene (*TERT*) are found in many human cancers (eg, melanoma, glioblastoma, hepatocellular carcinoma), including both NMIBC and MIBC.[2,27,41,42] Pietzak and colleagues[27] identified TERT promoter mutations in 61% of LGTa, 88% of HGTa, 79% of HGT1, and 85% of MSK-MIBC tumors without a significant difference across stage (*P* = .2) or grade (*P* = .15), with similar frequencies noted in other studies.[42] Given its high frequency of occurrence and persistence across various bladder cancer grades/stages, TERT may play a functional role in early bladder tumorigenesis.[42,43] A common polymorphism within the *TERT* promoter binding site acts as a modifier of the TERT mutation and affects survival and tumor recurrence.[42] In the absence of this variant allele polymorphism, patients with Tis, Ta, and T1 tumors bearing *TERT* mutations trended toward worse survival (HR, 2.19; 95% CI, 1.02–4.70) and higher risk of tumor recurrence (HR, 1.85; 95% CI, 1.11–3.08) compared with patients with the allele polymorphism present.[42] From a diagnostic standpoint, *TERT* promoter mutations are easily detected in voided urine and could aid in risk stratification of patients early in disease.[43,44]

Genomics of Tumor Progression

Although most patients diagnosed with bladder cancer are non–muscle invasive at presentation, ~15% to 20% of patients with NMIBC progress to muscle invasive (MIBC).[45] Studies have referred to these NMIBCs as progressors[39] or secondary MIBC.[46] Two of the candidate genes proposed in tumor progression are *E2F1* and *CDKN2A*. *E2F1* is a regulator of cell apoptosis and has been linked with tumor invasion and metastasis in multiple cancer types.[47] Microarray gene expression

profiling of 102 NMIBCs showed upregulation of *E2F1* and its downstream targets, *EZH2* and *SUZ12*, in patients with progression to muscle-invasive disease (*P*<.001).[48] Transfection of urothelial cells with a plasmid vector coding *E2F1*, *EZH2*, and *SUZ12* found that their expression correlated with increased proliferation, migration, invasiveness, and chemoresistance to mitomycin C and BCG.[48] CDK2NA is a cell cycle regulator involved in G1-S cell cycle arrest.[49] CDKN2A was found to be lost in the invasive portion of NMIBCs and our group identified loss of CDKN2A in 37% of T1s at progression compared with only 6% in nonprogressors (*P* = .10).[39,50] Only tumors with progression had both *TP53* and *CDK2NA* loss, suggesting that loss of both checkpoints in cell cycle progression may be necessary for progression.[39]

In a comparison of primary with secondary MIBC, the frequency of *ERCC2* mutations was significantly greater in primary MIBCs (11% vs 1.8%; *P* = .044), potentially resulting in decreased response to cisplatin chemotherapy (26% vs 45%; *P* = .02) and significantly worse recurrence-free, cancer-specific, and overall survival.[46] Whether *ERCC2* mutations are more common in primary MIBC, or loss of *ERCC2* mutations occurs during clonal selection and progression to MIBC is unknown. One hypothesis to explain the aggressive nature of secondary MIBC is that during progression TMB decreases to reduce the number of neoantigens, resulting in immune escape. Although more research is needed, insight into progression genomics is critical because patients with NMIBC with risk factors for progression may benefit from upfront cystectomy or enrollment in clinical trials rather than standard immunotherapies (eg, BCG) at the time of initial diagnosis.

PREDICTING RESPONSE TO BACILLUS CALMETTE-GUÉRIN

BCG is the most effective intravesical immunotherapy available for NMIBC to decrease recurrence (32.6%–42.1%), progression (9.5%–13.4%), and death from bladder cancer, but at least 40% of patients do not respond to BCG, and response decreases with age.[51] Tumor, host, and BCG factors are identified here that may aid in predicting BCG responsiveness and risk stratification before and while on BCG therapy. Known clinicopathologic factors that predict recurrence after BCG therapy include female sex, tumor multiplicity, and presence of CIS, whereas high-grade disorder, T1 tumors, and early recurrence on 3-month endoscopic evaluation predict progression to MIBC.[52] Upfront limitations in overall BCG data interpretation include differences in BCG strains; maintenance BCG protocol; and definitions of clinical response, recurrence, progression, and failure.

Tumor Factors

Neoantigens

Self-antigens are expressed by both tumor and normal cells, which leads to tolerance by the immune system to these antigens. Neoantigens derived from mutated proteins are specific to cancer cells only, which limits tolerance, promotes immune cell infiltration, and makes these proteins attractive candidates for immunotherapy targets.[53] Neoantigens are prognostic and are associated with overall survival in MIBC. In lung cancer and melanoma, tumor responsiveness to immune checkpoint inhibitors is directly correlated with increased TMB and neoantigen load, with the top 20% of TMB being more likely to respond.[54–56] Thus, tumors with a low TMB may have a decreased response to BCG.[57] Our group showed a significant decrease in TMB and thus neoantigen load in patients who progressed on BCG or had

metastatic disease compared with nonprogressors ($P = .02$).[39] In a comparison of 35 NMIBCs treated with BCG (17 responsive and 18 unresponsive), the median TMB was 3 mutations per mutation burden (MB), with a significant difference noted in responsiveness (4.9 mutations per MB vs 2.8 mutations per MB; $P = .017$). Tumors with a high TMB (>3 mutations per MB) were associated with a greater response to BCG (71% vs 28%; $P = .01$). Higher TMB was associated with longer recurrence-free survival (38 vs 15 months; $P = .0092$).[39] Furthermore, loss of TMB was most recently found in the PURE-01 cohort in tumors that progressed.[58] These findings suggest that increased TMB may be predictive of responsiveness to BCG, and this possibility continues to be investigated.

Genomics of bacillus Calmette-Guérin responsiveness

Genetic features associated with BCG response is an active area of research. **Table 1** summarizes current knowledge regarding specific genes associated with BCG responsiveness in NMIBC. Ke and colleagues[59] found that certain

Table 1
Genomics of predicting bacillus Calmette-Guérin responsiveness

Study, Year	Study Design	Number of Patients	Sample	Stage/ Grade Tumor	Genomic Markers Assessed	Results
Ke et al,[59] 2015	Prospective	191	Blood	Ta, T1, CIS	SNPs: glutathione pathway genes	Predictor of recurrence after BCG: rs7265992 in *GSS* gene
Meeks et al,[39] 2016	Retrospective	25	Tissue	HGTa, HGT1, CIS	*CDK2NA*, TMB	Predictor of progression after BCG: loss of *CDK2NA*, TMB
Pietzak et al,[27] 2017	Prospective	62	Tissue	Ta, T1, CIS	341-gene panel	Predictor of recurrence after BCG: *ARID1A* mutation
Lima et al,[60] 2015	Retrospective	204	Blood	Ta, T1, CIS	PMs in immune response genes	Prediction score based on clinicopathologic factors and immune response PMs
Kim et al,[61] 2010	Retrospective	80	Tissue	T1	424 and 287 genes predictive of recurrence and progression	Gene signatures predictive of recurrence (12 total) and progression (12 total)

Abbreviations: PMs, polymorphisms; SNPs, single nucleotide polymorphisms.

glutathione (GSH) pathway genomic variations could predict recurrence after BCG. GSH is involved in cellular antioxidation and detoxification as well as T-cell and neutrophil function and survival. In 191 patients with NMIBC who underwent BCG therapy (induction ± maintenance), recurrence after BCG was significantly associated with polymorphism rs7265992 in GSH synthetase (GSS).[59] As discussed earlier, our group found that in 10 patients with high-risk NMIBC treated with BCG, predictors of progression to MIBC included high TMB and loss of CDK2NA.[39] Pietzak and colleagues[27] found ARID1A mutation (a chromatin-modifying gene) was significantly associated with increased risk of recurrence (HR, 3.14; 95% CI, 1.51–6.51; P = .002) after BCG induction in 62 patients with high-grade NMIBC. Lima and colleagues[60] developed a BCG responsiveness predictive score using clinicopathologic factors as well as immune system gene polymorphisms from genotyping serum of 204 patients with NMIBC treated with BCG (single nucleotide polymorphisms in tumor necrosis factor α [TNFA]-1031T/C [rs1799964], interleukin [IL] 2 receptor α [IL2RA] rs2104286 T/C, IL17A-197G/A [rs2275913], IL17RA-809A/G [rs4819554], IL18R1 rs3771171 T/C, intercellular adhesion molecule 1 [ICAM-1] K469E [rs5498], Fas ligand [FASL]-844T/C [rs763110], and tumor necrosis factor [TNF]-related apoptosis-inducing ligand receptor 1 [TRAILR1]-397T/G [rs79037040]). In addition, Kim and colleagues[61] identified 424 and 287 genes that were significantly associated with recurrence and progression-free survival, respectively, in 80 T1 patients after BCG therapy. From these, they identified gene signatures predictive of recurrence (12 total; HR, 3.38; P = .048) and progression (12 total; HR, 10.49; P = .048) (see Table 1).

Host Factors (Tumor Microenvironment and Immune Response)

The tumor microenvironment (TME) is composed of cancer cells, stroma (immune cells, cytokines, fibroblasts, mesenchymal cells, vasculature), and extracellular matrix. The complex interplay between these cell types and signaling molecules underlies tumorigenesis, growth, and metastasis.[62] Although the exact mechanism of BCG is still unknown, it must intercalate into the TME and increase the immunogenicity of bladder cancer antigens. Thus, variable amounts of stroma density may affect BCG response (Fig. 2A). It is thought that BCG is internalized by urothelial cells, processed and presented to BCG-specific CD4+ T cells, and induces a T-helper (Th) 1--directed

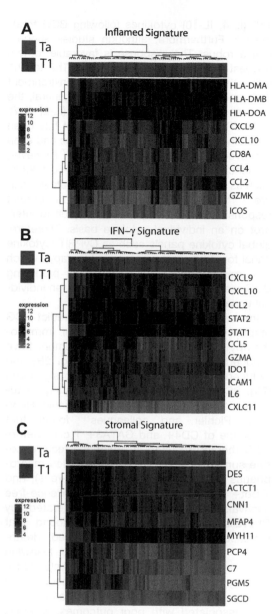

Fig. 2. Immune-related and stromal-related gene expression in Ta (red) and T1 (blue) tumors before BCG therapy. (A) Immune signature, (B) interferon (IFN)-γ signature, (C) stromal gene expression. Lower-stage tumors have fewer T cells or inflamed signatures at diagnosis, with relatively low IFN expression. Inflamed tumors tend to be higher stage but also have increased stromal signature that can impede immune cell infiltration.

influx of macrophages, cluster of differentiation (CD) 8+ T cells, and natural killer (NK) cells to destroy tumor cells.[63] The role of the Th1 versus Th2 dichotomy in BCG responsiveness is complex because patients show both increased Th1 (IL-1, IL-2, IL-6, IL-8, IL-12, TNF, interferon [IFN]-γ and

Th2 (IL-4, IL-10) cytokines following BCG treatment.[52] Furthermore, although studies suggest that a robust Th1 response is favorable, others suggest it is the conversion from a Th2 to Th1 rather than an already polarized Th1 environment that predicts responsiveness.[51,64] In general, the presence of Th1 urinary cytokines (IL-2, IL-8, IL-12, TNF) early after BCG treatment has been predictive of a favorable BCG response and even improved cancer-specific survival.[65–67] However, presence of Th2 immunosuppressive cytokines such as IL-10 does not foreshadow treatment failure.[51,68,69] The optimal cytokine milieu to predict responsiveness is complex and difficult to interpret on an individual cytokine basis. Therefore, global cytokine panels such as CyPRIT (cytokine panel for response to intravesical therapy), which is currently undergoing validation in predicting BCG response, may be more helpful than individual urinary cytokines in the future.[51,69]

Immune cell infiltration may also predict BCG response, similar to other forms of immunotherapy. Before BCG therapy, Ta tumors have reduced baseline T-cell infiltrate (**Fig. 2**B) and reduced STAT1 signaling (IFN-γ signature) (**Fig. 2**C) compared with T1, suggesting Ta tumors may be "cold" or less immunogenic. However, Pichler and colleagues[70] found that presence of CD4+ and GATA3+ T cells before BCG therapy resulted in prolonged recurrence-free survival, whereas tumor-associated macrophages (TAMs), T-regulatory cells (T-regs), and T-bet+ T cells indicated shorter recurrence-free survival. These findings were reiterated by Chevalier and colleagues,[71] who found that increased infiltration of programmed death-ligand 1 (PD-L1)–expressing T-regs following BCG predicted tumor recurrence. A systemic review by Kamat and colleagues[51] further showed that the presence of CD68+ TAMs and T-regs was associated with poor outcomes, whereas M1 macrophages (Th1-associated macrophages), NK cells, and CD4+ T-cell infiltration were predictive of enhanced response.

Bacillus Calmette-Guérin Factors

To add to the complexity of predicting response to BCG therapy, there are multiple BCG strains, doses, and protocols used by providers worldwide.[72] Since its release in 1921, multiple BCG strains have been cultivated and accumulated mutations leading to differences in efficacy. There are more than 8 strains currently available, although BCG Connaught and BCG Tice were historically the most common used in the United States and Europe.[73] Rentsch and colleagues[73] compared the efficacy of BCG Connaught and BCG Tice in a prospective trial of 142 patients with high-risk NMIBC. Five-year recurrence-free survival was significantly greater for BCG Connaught compared with BCG Tice (74% vs 48%; $P = .0108$), whereas 5-year progression-free, overall, and disease-specific survival were comparable. Using a mouse model as well, the investigators found BCG Connaught induced greater priming of BCG-specific CD8+ T cells and enhanced recruitment of T cells to bladder and regional lymph nodes compared with BCG Tice. Because of closure of the Sanofi laboratories, BCG Connaught is no longer available in the United States, Canada, United Kingdom, or France. US patients are currently receive BCG Tice through Merck, which has another foreseen shortage in 2019.[72] In light of past and likely future shortages, it is important to identify other viable strains and ways to reduce number of BCG doses. SWOG 1602 aims to compare BCG Tice with BCG Tokyo-172 strain with and without priming vaccination to see whether the strains have comparable efficacy and whether prior inoculation enhances responsiveness to BCG (NCT03091660).

INVESTIGATIONAL, NON–BACILLUS CALMETTE-GUÉRIN–BASED THERAPIES

Given shortages as well as variable patient response rates to BCG, it is important to identify other treatments for NMIBC that reduce recurrence and progression to muscle-invasive disease. Non–BCG-based therapies currently under investigation are discussed here.

Programmed Cell Death Protein 1/ Programmed Death-Ligand 1 Checkpoint Inhibitors

PD-L1 is expressed on antigen-presenting and tumor cells. When bound to programmed cell death protein 1 (PD-1) on T cells, this interaction causes T-cell inactivation. Therefore, antibody blockade of PD-L1 (atezolizumab, durvalumab, avelumab) or PD-1 (pembrolizumab, nivolumab) improves T-cell activation and antitumor immunity. Increased PD-L1 expression has been linked to poor response to BCG, increasing tumor stage (7% Ta, 16% T1, 23% T2, 30% T3/4, 45% CIS and high-grade tumors (odds ratio, 2.4; $P = .009$).[74] Furthermore, PD-L1 expression is not fixed but changes over the lifetime of the tumor and with response to treatment.[74] In addition, a complex interplay between the TME and tumor affects responsiveness to PD-L1 blockade. In MIBC (TCGA dataset), Wang and colleagues[75] showed that tumors with high T-cell infiltration and stromal-related gene expression have lower response rates, progression-free survival, and overall survival with PD-1 blockade (nivolumab). Although this is still under investigation in NMIBC, **Fig. 2** suggests that TME, immune cell infiltration, and stromal gene expression variations exist between Ta and T1 tumors and could affect responsiveness to PD-1/PD-L1 targeting therapies. Although there is no long-term evidence for the efficacy of checkpoint inhibitors in NMIBC, checkpoint inhibitors have shown clinical benefit in MIBC and metastatic patients (IMVIGOR211, KEYNOTE045) and trials in non–muscle-invasive disease are currently underway.[76,77]

SUMMARY

NMIBC is heterogeneous, but current diagnostic and treatment strategies rely primarily on clinical parameters, lacking individualization to tumor and host biology. Advances in sequencing technology, insight into differential BCG responses, and new investigational treatment targets will soon offer clinicians new, precision-based tools to risk stratify and determine treatment regimens for future patients with bladder cancer.

REFERENCES

1. Meeks JJ, Lerner SP. Molecular landscape of non-muscle invasive bladder cancer. Cancer Cell 2017; 32:550–1.
2. Hurst CD, Alder O, Platt FM, et al. Genomic subtypes of non-invasive bladder cancer with distinct metabolic profile, clinical outcome, and female gender bias in KMD2A mutation frequency. Cancer Cell 2017;32(5):701–15.
3. Cancer Genome Atlas Network. Comprehensive molecular characterization of urothelial bladder carcinoma. Nature 2014;507(7492):315–22.
4. Robertson AG, Kim J, Al-Ahmadie H, et al. Comprehensive molecular characterization of muscle-invasive bladder cancer. Cell 2017;171(3):540–56.
5. Biton A, Bernand-Pierrot I, Lou Y, et al. Independent component analysis uncovers the landscape of the bladder tumor transcriptome and reveals insights into luminal and basal subtypes. Cell Rep 2014; 9(4):1235–45.
6. El Behi M, Krumeich S, Lodilinsky C, et al. An essential role for decorin in bladder cancer invasiveness. EMBO Mol Med 2013;5(12):1835–51.
7. Glaser AP, Fantini D, Shilatifard A, et al. The evolving genomic landscape of urothelial carcinoma. Nat Rev Urol 2017;14(4):213–29.
8. Lawrence MS, Stojanov P, Polak P, et al. Mutational heterogeneity in cancer and the search for new cancer-associated genes. Nature 2013;499(7457):214–8.
9. Glaser AP, Fantini D, Wang Y, et al. APOBEC-mediated mutagenesis in urothelial carcinoma is associated with improved survival, mutations in DNA damage response genes, and immune response. Oncotarget 2017;9(4):4537–48.
10. Hedegaard J, Lamy P, Nordentoft I, et al. Comprehensive transcriptional analysis of early-stage urothelial carcinoma. Cancer Cell 2016;30:27–42.
11. Lamy P, Nordentoft I, Birkenkamp-Demtroder K, et al. Paired exome analysis reveals clonal evolution and potential therapeutic targets in urothelial carcinoma. Cancer Res 2016;76:5894–906.
12. Nordentoft I, Lamy P, Birkenkamp-Demtroder K, et al. Mutational context and diverse clonal development in early and late bladder cancer. Cell Rep 2014;7:1649–63.
13. Hurst CD, Platt FM, Taylor CF, et al. Novel tumor subgroups of urothelial carcinoma of the bladder defined by integrated genomic analysis. Clin Cancer Res 2012;18:5865–77.
14. Blaveri E, Brewer JL, Roydasgupta R, et al. Bladder cancer stage and outcome by array-based comparative genomic hybridization. Clin Cancer Res 2005; 11:7012–22.
15. Granberg-Ohman I, Tribukait B, Wijkstrom H. Cytogenetic analysis of 62 transitional cell bladder carcinomas. Cancer Genet Cytogenet 1984;11:69–85.
16. Richter J, Jiang F, Gorog JP, et al. Marked genetic differences between stage pTa and stage pT1 papillary bladder cancer detected by comparative genomic hybridization. Cancer Res 1997;57:2860–4.
17. Hurst CD, Knowles MA. Mutational landscape of non-muscle-invasive bladder cancer. Urol Oncol 2018;S1078-1439(18):30398–403.
18. Rampias T, Vgenopoulou P, Avgeris M, et al. A new tumor suppressor role for the Notch pathway in bladder cancer. Nat Med 2014;20:1199–205.
19. Griefe A, Jankowiak S, Steinbring J, et al. Canonical Notch signaling is inactive in urothelial carcinoma. BMC Cancer 2014;14:628–41.
20. Maraver A, Fernandez-Marcos PJ, Cash TP, et al. NOTCH pathway inactivation promotes bladder cancer progression. J Clin Invest 2015;125(2):824–30.
21. Iyer G, Hanrahan AJ, Milowsky MI, et al. Genome sequencing identifies a basis for everolimus sensitivity. Science 2012;228(6104):221–3.
22. Svatek RS, Ji N, de Leon E, et al. Rapamycin prevents surgery-induced immune dysfunction in patients with bladder cancer. Cancer Immunol Res 2018. https://doi.org/10.1158/2326-6066.CIR-18-0336.
23. Billerey C, Chopin D, Aubriot-Lorton MH, et al. Frequent FGFR3 mutations in papillary non-

invasive bladder (pTa) tumors. Am J Pathol 2001; 158:1955–9.

24. Kimura T, Suzuki H, Ohashi T, et al. The incidence of thanatophoric dysplasia mutations in FGFR3 gene is higher in low-grade or superficial bladder carcinomas. Cancer 2001;92:2555–61.

25. Tomlinson D, Baldo O, Harnden P, et al. FGFR3 protein expression and its relationship to mutation status and prognostic variables in bladder cancer. J Pathol 2007;213:91–8.

26. Hernandez S, Lopez-Knowles E, Lloreta J, et al. Prospective study of FGFR3 mutations as a prognostic factor in nonmuscle invasive urothelial bladder carcinomas. J Clin Oncol 2006;24:3664–71.

27. Pietzak EJ, Bagrodia A, Cha EK, et al. Next-generation sequencing of nonmuscle invasive bladder cancer reveals potential biomarkers and rational therapeutic targets. Eur Urol 2017;72(6):952–9.

28. Liu X, Zhang W, Geng D, et al. Clinical significance of fibroblast growth factor receptor-3 mutations in bladder cancer: a systemic review and meta-analysis. Genet Mol Res 2014;13(1):1109–20.

29. Guo G, Sun X, Chen C, et al. Whole-genome and whole-exome sequencing of bladder cancer identifies alteration in genes involved in sister chromatid cohesion and segregation. Nat Genet 2013;45(12): 1459–63.

30. Williams SV, Hurst CD, Knowles MA. Oncogenic FGFR3 gene fusions in bladder cancer. Hum Mol Genet 2013;22:795–803.

31. Hahn NM, Bivalacqua TJ, Ross AE, et al. A phase II trial of dovitinib in BCG-unresponsive urothelial carcinoma with FGFR3 mutations or overexpression: Hoosier cancer research network trial HCRN 12-157. Clin Cancer Res 2017;23(12):3003–11.

32. Siefker-Radtke A, Necchi A, Park SH, et al. First results from the primary analysis population of the phase 2 study of erdafitinib (ERDA;JNJ-42756493) in patients (pts) with metastatic or unresectable urothelial carcinoma (mUC) and FGFR alterations (FGFRalt). Available at: https://ascopubs.org/doi/abs/10.1200/JCO.2018.36.15_suppl.4503. Accessed March 1, 2019.

33. Pal SK, Rosenberg JE, Hoffman-Censits JH, et al. Efficacy of BGJ398, a fibroblast growth factor receptor 1-3 inhibitor, in patients with previously treated advanced urothelial carcinoma with FGFR3 alterations. Cancer Discov 2018;8(7):812–21.

34. Moasser MM. The oncogene HER2: its signaling and transforming functions and its role in human cancer pathogenesis. Oncogene 2007;26(45):6469–87.

35. Kiss B, Wyatt AW, Douglas J, et al. Her2 alterations in muscle-invasive bladder cancer: Patient selection beyond protein expression for targeted therapy. Sci Rep 2017;7:42713.

36. Chen PC, Yu HJ, Chang YH, et al. Her2 amplification distinguishes a subset of non-muscle invasive bladder cancers with a high risk of progression. J Clin Pathol 2013;66(2):113–9.

37. Breyer J, Otto W, Wirtz RM, et al. ERBB2 expression as potential risk-stratification for early cystectomy in patients with pT1 bladder cancer and concomitant carcinoma in situ. Urol Int 2017;98:282–9.

38. Lopez-Knowles E, Hernandez S, Malats N, et al. PIK3CA mutations are an early genetic alteration associated with FGFR3 mutations in superficial papillary bladder tumors. Cancer Res 2006;66: 7401–4.

39. Meeks JJ, Carneiro BA, Pai SG, et al. Genomic characterization of high risk non-muscle invasive bladder cancer. Oncotarget 2016;7(46):75176–84.

40. Ler LD, Ghosh S, Chai X, et al. Loss of tumor suppressor KDM6A amplifies PRC2-regulated transcriptional repression in bladder cancer and can be targeted through inhibition of EZH2. Sci Transl Med 2017;9(378) [pii:eaai8312].

41. Bell RJA, Rube HT, Xavier-Magalhaes A, et al. Understanding TERT promoter mutations: a common path to immortality. Mol Cancer Res 2017;14(4): 315–23.

42. Rachakonda PS, Hosen I, de Verdier PJ, et al. TERT promoter mutations in bladder cancer affect patient survival and disease recurrence through modification by a common polymorphism. Proc Natl Acad Sci U S A 2013;110:17426–31.

43. Kinde I, Munari E, Faraj SF, et al. TERT promoter mutations occur early in urothelial neoplasia and are biomarkers of early disease and disease recurrence in urine. Cancer Res 2013;73:7162–7.

44. Hurst CD, Platt FM, Knowles MA. Comprehensive mutation analysis of the TERT promoter in bladder cancer and detection of mutations in voided urine. Eur Urol 2014;65:367–9.

45. Chamie K, Litwin MS, Bassett JC, et al. Recurrence of high-risk bladder cancer: a population-based analysis. Cancer 2013;119(17):3219–27.

46. Pietzak EJ, Zabor EC, Bagrodia A, et al. Genomic differences between "primary" and "secondary" muscle-invasive bladder cancer as a basis for disparate outcomes to cisplatin-based neoadjuvant chemotherapy. Eur Urol 2019;75(2):231–9.

47. Putzer B, Engelmann D. E2F1 apoptosis counterattacked: evil strikes back. Trends Mol Med 2013; 19(2):89–98.

48. Lee SR, Roh YG, Kim SK, et al. Activation of EZH2 and SUZ12 regulated by E2F1 predicts disease progression and aggressive characteristics of bladder cancer. Clin Cancer Res 2015;21(23):5391–403.

49. Sherr CJ, McCornick F. The RB and p53 pathways in cancer. Cancer Cell 2002;2(2):103–12.

50. Warrick JI, Hovelson DH, Amin A, et al. Tumor evolution and progression in multifocal and paired non-invasive/invasive urothelial carcinoma. Virchows Arch 2015;466(3):297–311.

51. Kamat AM, Li R, O'Donnell MA, et al. Predicting response to intravesical bacillus calmette-guerin immunotherapy: are we there yet? A systemic review. Eur Urol 2018;73:738–48.

52. Fernandez-Gomez J, Solsona E, Unda M, et al. Prognostic factors in patients with non-muscle-invasive bladder cancer treated with bacillus Calmette-Guerin: multivariate analysis of data from four randomized CUETO trials. Eur Urol 2008; 53(5):992–1001.

53. Efremova M, Finotello F, Rieder D, et al. Neoantigens generated by individual mutations and their role in cancer immunity and immunotherapy. Front Immunol 2017;8:1679–87.

54. Rizvi NA, Hellmann MD, Snyder A, et al. Cancer immunology. Mutational landscape determines sensitivity to PD-1 blockade in non-small cell lung cancer. Science 2015;348:124–8.

55. Van Allen EM, Miao D, Schilling B, et al. Genomic correlates of response to CTLA-4 blockade in metastatic melanoma. Science 2015;350:207–11.

56. Le DT, Uram JN, Wang H, et al. PD-1 blockade in tumors with mismatch-repair deficiency. N Engl J Med 2015;372:2509–20.

57. Samstein RM, Lee CH, Shoushtari AN, et al. Tumor mutational load predicts survival after immunotherapy across multiple cancer types. Nat Genet 2019;51(2):202–6.

58. Necchi A, Anichini A, Raggi D, et al. Pembrolizumab as neoadjuvant therapy before radical cystectomy in patients with muscle invasive urothelial bladder carcinoma (PURE-01): an open-label, single-arm, phase II study. J Clin Oncol 2018. https://doi.org/10.1200/JCO.18.01148.

59. Ke HL, Lin J, Ye Y, et al. Genetic variations in glutathione pathway genes predict cancer recurrence in patients treated with transurethral resection and bacillus calmette-guerin instillation for non-muscle invasive bladder cancer. Ann Surg Oncol 2015; 22(12):4104–10.

60. Lima L, Oliveira D, Ferreira JA, et al. The role of functional polymorphisms in immune response genes as biomarkers of bacille Calmette-Guérin (BCG) immunotherapy outcome in bladder cancer: establishment of a predictive profile in a Southern Europe population. BJU Int 2015; 116(5):753–63.

61. Kim YJ, Ha YS, Kim SK, et al. Gene signatures for the prediction of bacillus calmette-guerin immunotherapy in primary pT1 bladder cancers. Clin Cancer Res 2010;16(7):2131–7.

62. Kang HW, Kim WJ, Yun SJ. The role of the tumor microenvironment in bladder cancer development and progression. Transl Cancer Res 2017;6: S744–58.

63. Miyake M, Tatsumi Y, Gotoh D, et al. Regulatory T cells and tumor-associated macrophages in the tumor microenvironment in non-muscle invasive bladder cancer treated with intravesical bacille Calmette-Guérin: a long-term follow-up study of a Japanese cohort. Int J Mol Sci 2017;18(10): 2186–98.

64. Nunez-Nateras R, Castle EP, Protheroe CA, et al. Predicting response to bacillus Calmette-Guerin (BCG) in patients with carcinoma in situ of the bladder. Urol Oncol 2014;32(1):e23–30.

65. Thalmann GN, Sermier A, Rentsch C, et al. Urinary Interleukin-8 and 18 predict the response of superficial bladder cancer to intravesical therapy with bacillus Calmette-Guerin. J Urol 2000;164: 2129–33.

66. Shintani Y, Sawada Y, Inagaki T, et al. Intravesical instillation therapy with bacillus Calmette-Guerin for superficial bladder cancer: study of the mechanism of bacillus Calmette-Guerin immunotherapy. Int J Urol 2007;14:140–6.

67. Pichler R, Gruenbacher G, Culig Z, et al. Intratumoral Th2 predisposition combines with an increased Th1 functional phenotype in clinical response to intravesical BCG in bladder cancer. Cancer Immunol Immunother 2017;66:427–40.

68. Nadler R, Luo Y, Zhao W, et al. Interleukin 10 induced augmentation of delayed-type hypersensitivity (DTH) enhances Mycobacterium bovis bacillus Calmette-Guerin (BCG) mediated antitumour activity. Clin Exp Immunol 2003;131:206–16.

69. Kamat AM, Briggman J, Urbauer DL, et al. Cytokine panel for response to intravesical therapy (CyPRIT) nomogram of changes in urinary cytokine levels predicts patient response to bacillus Calmette-Guerin. Eur Urol 2016;69(2):197–200.

70. Pichler R, Fritz J, Zavadil C, et al. Tumor-infiltrating immune cell subpopulations influence the oncologic outcome after intravesical bacillus Calmette-Guerin therapy in bladder cancer. Oncotarget 2016;7: 39916–30.

71. Chevalier MF, Schneider AK, Cesson V, et al. Conventional and PD-L1-expressing regulatory T cells are enriched during BCG therapy and may limit its efficacy. Eur Urol 2018;74(5):540–4.

72. Bandari J, Maganty A, MacLeod LC, et al. Manufacturing and the market: Rationalizing the shortage of bacillus Calmette-Guérin. Eur Urol 2018;4(4):481–4.

73. Rentsch CA, Birkhauser FD, Biot C, et al. Bacillus Calmette-Guérin strain differences have an impact on clinical outcome in bladder cancer immunotherapy. Eur Urol 2014;66(4):677–88.

74. Inman BA, Sebo TJ, Frigola X, et al. PD-L1 (B7-H1) expression by urothelial carcinoma of the bladder and BCG-induced gramulomata. Cancer 2007; 109(8):1499–505.

75. Wang L, Saci A, Szabo PM, et al. EMT- and stroma-related gene expression and resistance to PD-1

blockade in urothelial cancer. Nat Commun 2018; 9(1):3503–15.

76. Powles T, Duran I, van der Heijden MS, et al. Atezolizumab versus chemotherapy in patients with platinum-treated locally advanced or metastatic urothelial carcinoma (IMvigor211): a multicenter, open-label, phase 3 randomised controlled trial. Lancet 2018;391(10122):748–57.

77. Bellmunt J, de Wit R, Vaughn DJ, et al. Pembrolizumab as second-line therapy for advanced urothelial carcinoma. N Engl J Med 2017;376: 1015–26.

Salvage Therapy Using Bacillus Calmette-Guérin Derivatives or Single Agent Chemotherapy

Christopher R. Haas, MD*, James M. McKiernan, MD

KEYWORDS

- Salvage intravesical chemotherapy • Gemcitabine • Docetaxel • BCG derivatives • BCG failure

KEY POINTS

- Patients with Bacillus Calmette-Guérin–unresponsive disease who refuse or are ineligible for cystectomy remain a challenging patient population to treat without a gold standard treatment.
- Studies of single-agent chemotherapy with valrubicin, gemcitabine, and docetaxel in the salvage setting after Bacillus Calmette-Guérin failure have demonstrated moderate efficacy at a cost of slightly increased oncologic risk.
- Bacillus Calmette-Guérin derivates such as mycobacterial cell wall nucleic acid complex achieved response rates comparable with single-agent intravesical chemotherapy in the salvage setting; however, disease progression was fairly high.

INTRODUCTION TO SALVAGE INTRAVESICAL THERAPIES

Patients who have high-grade recurrences after intravesical Bacillus Calmette-Guérin (BCG) represent a particularly challenging disease state to manage. Radical cystectomy (RC) remains the oncologic gold standard in patients at high risk of recurrence after BCG failure in non–muscle-invasive bladder cancer (NMIBC); however, the significant morbidity of this operation makes some patients ineligible and others highly desirous of a bladder sparing approach. The term salvage therapy implies an attempt to salvage the patient's bladder in lieu of undergoing a radical cystectomy. Historically, the majority of trials testing salvage intravesical therapies have been single-arm trials that have enrolled patients with varying degrees of prior exposure to BCG and varying degrees of pathologic risk, making direct comparisons of efficacy between agents very difficult. Therefore, when assessing the efficacy of the various salvage agents presented in the following articles, the reported recurrence and progression-free survival rates must be tempered with knowledge of the initial disease severity and prior BCG exposure of patients included in the trials. With this in mind, overall 1- to 2-year recurrence-free survival (RFS) rates of various agents are modest ranging from 18% to 43%.[1]

In an effort to clarify and simplify BCG failure for ease of comparison across trials and to identify appropriate eligibility criteria for novel salvage intravesical therapies, Kamat and colleagues[1] suggested that new trials investigating salvage intravesical therapy primarily include BCG-unresponsive patients, with a further breakdown of the proportion of patients who fit into

Disclosure Statement: The authors have nothing to disclose.
Columbia University Department of Urology, Herbert Irving Pavilion, 161 Fort Washington Avenue, 11th Floor, New York, NY 10032, USA
* Corresponding author.
E-mail address: crh2109@cumc.columbia.edu

Urol Clin N Am 47 (2020) 47–54
https://doi.org/10.1016/j.ucl.2019.09.007

BCG-refractory, -relapsing, and -intolerant categories. BCG-unresponsive disease combines BCG-refractory and BCG-relapsing disease to provide the urologist a clear definition for when further intravesical BCG is unlikely to provide benefit. For the purposes of being considered as BCG unresponsive, BCG-relapsing patients must have a high-grade recurrence within 6 months of achieving a disease-free state after 2 induction courses of BCG or high-grade recurrence after induction plus maintenance. Numerous studies have found that earlier high-risk recurrences after BCG carry a higher risk of progression, with salvage intravesical therapies having poor success rates in this setting.[2,3] As detailed more extensively in the Russell E.N. Becker and colleagues' article in this issue, "Identification of Candidates for Salvage Therapy: The Past, Present, and Future of Defining BCG Failure," BCG-refractory disease is composed of persistent high-grade NMIBC at 6 months despite adequate BCG treatment. Although intermediate-or high-risk patients with persistent or recurrent Ta disease or carcinoma in situ (CIS) after a single course of induction BCG may benefit from an additional induction course of BCG, patients with high-grade T1 disease after a single BCG induction course are also deemed BCG refractory and should be offered radical cystectomy as a gold standard.[4]

Should patients either be unfit for radical cystectomy or refuse cystectomy after demonstrating BCG-unresponsive disease, we recommend that the patient enroll in clinical trials if able because no single or combined agent has demonstrated clear superiority in the salvage setting. In this article, we detail prior studies of salvage therapy using a single agent intravesical chemotherapy or BCG derivatives with the aim of giving the reader a sense of their comparable efficacy by looking at outcomes in the context of their often heterogenous treatment populations (**Table 1**).

MITOMYCIN C

Mitomycin C (MMC), an alkylating agent that cross-links DNA and has been in use since 1974,[5] has been among the most extensively used intravesical chemotherapeutic agents in bladder cancer. The vast majority of studies investigated MMC as a first line alternative to BCG or in the immediate single-dose postoperative setting. There have been roughly 9 randomized controlled trials since the early 1990s comparing first-line induction MMC versus BCG in the various NMIBC risk groups. Several metanalyses have come to slightly different conclusions ranging from BCG's superiority regardless of risk group,[6] to the

Cochrane's group conclusion of BCG superiority only in the high-risk subgroup,[7] to a more recent meta-analysis using individual patient data finding BCG superiority only when maintenance therapy was used.[8] Synthesizing our current knowledge of the data, both American Urological Association[4] and European Association of Urology[9] guidelines recommend BCG as the superior choice for first-line intravesical therapy in high-risk NMIBC, whereas both MMC and BCG remain viable options in intermediate risk disease with risk–benefit tradeoffs depending on the spectrum of disease and patient. Studies investigating MMC in the salvage setting involve either the use of MMC in combination (sequential or alternating) with BCG or other intravesical therapies, or use of MMC with enhanced delivery systems, such as electromotive devices or hyperthermia, and are thus left for discussion in subsequent articles.

VALRUBICIN

Valrubicin is notable for being the only US Food and Drug Administration (FDA)-approved intravesical medication specifically for BCG-unresponsive CIS. It is a semisynthetic analog of the anthracycline doxorubicin that primarily affects nucleic acid metabolism.[10] Despite its FDA approval, this agent is infrequently used because of its unimpressive long-term results and poor tolerability. The pivotal study in the year 2000 by Steinberg and colleagues[11] that garnered FDA approval was a single-arm 90 patient phase I/II trial that enrolled patients with CIS who had had at least 1 prior induction course of BCG with or without maintenance. Seventeen percent of patients had concomitant papillary tumors before first instillation that were completely resected, and 70% of patients had at least 2 prior BCG induction courses, representing a high-risk cohort overall. They found a 21% complete response (CR) rate at 6 months, of which only 7 (8%) remained disease free at the end a median follow-up of 30 months. The authors noted a significant portion of patients (56%) who underwent cystectomy at a median time of 20 months in the nonresponder group. They did not give a complete breakdown of final pathology, noting only that 15% of patients had stage pT3 or greater. Significant local toxicity was noted with 90% of patients experiencing at least one adverse event and 3 patients halting the induction course midway because of severe bladder symptoms.

Owing to a lapse in valrubicin production, it was not until 2009 with its reintroduction into the market that further patients could be recruited for an additional phase III trial of valrubicin. Dinney and colleagues[12] combined updated long-term follow-up data from the initial pivotal trial by Steinberg and colleagues,[11] while also recruiting an additional 80 patients with CIS who either failed BCG, were BCG intolerant, or had contraindications to BCG. As a result of this looser inclusion criteria, this trial was notable for having fewer patients meeting today's criteria for BCG unresponsive status as only 39% of patients had received 2 or more previous induction courses of BCG. Defining a CR as no evidence of disease on biopsy or cytology at the 6-month mark, the study found that both the new patients and updated results of the prior pivotal trial had a CR of 18%. Importantly, this study also found a long-term durability of only 10% at 1 year and only 4% at 2 years for the newly recruited patients, despite having 61% of patients who had only received 1 prior BCG induction. Furthermore, treatment with valrubicin was more irritative than most other agents with 86% of patients experiencing 1 or more local bladder symptom of either frequency, dysuria, and urinary urgency.[12] Because of the poor response rates and durability of response with significant local symptoms compared with other intravesical therapies, valrubicin is rarely used as a viable salvage option for patients.

GEMCITABINE

Gemcitabine and the taxane class of chemotherapy have been the most widely studied intravesical cytotoxic agents in the salvage setting and have demonstrated moderate efficacy. Gemcitabine, an inhibitor of DNA synthesis, is an agent commonly used in systemic chemotherapy for muscle invasive bladder cancer, and has recently seen an increase in its use in the single postoperative dose setting[13] and in combined regimens. As a solitary salvage intravesical agent, gemcitabine was first investigated in a phase II trial by Dalbagni and the MSKCC group.[14] They enrolled 30 patients who were deemed to be BCG refractory or BCG intolerant (3 patients), with 43% of patients having had 2 or more prior induction courses of BCG. 50% of patients initially achieved a CR; however, longer follow-up showed limited durability with 12 of 14 patients ultimately recurring for a 1-year RFS of 21%. The progression and cystectomy rates at 1 year were 3.5% and 20.5%, respectively.

Following up on the moderate success of Dalbagni and colleagues, Di Lorenzo and colleagues[15] conducted a randomized controlled trial of gemcitabine versus a second BCG induction for the treatment of recurrent disease after initial BCG induction. They enrolled 80 patients

with 40 patients in each group who were well-balanced in baseline characteristics; however, 30% of patients were classified as having low-grade disease and, therefore, would not be considered as high-risk BCG unresponsive disease after just 1 BCG induction course by most definitions. After a median follow-up of 15.5 months, the authors surprisingly found gemcitabine to have a significantly improved RFS rate compared with a second induction course of BCG (1 year, 55% vs 27%; P<.008). Despite an improved disease-free rate, other outcomes such as progression-free survival did not differ between groups, and in fact were quite high at 33% and 37.5% in the gemcitabine and BCG groups, respectively. The study authors attributed this finding to their particularly high-risk cohort, which is not supported by their presented baseline characteristics, but perhaps owing to understaging or undergrading of their cohort.

More recently in 2013, the SWOG S0353 phase II trial of intravesical gemcitabine enrolled 58 patients who all had recurrence after at least 2 prior induction courses of BCG that had been received up to 3 years before study enrollment (median time from last BCG was 205 days).[16] Eighty-nine percent of patients had high-risk disease at the time of enrollment. They found an initial 3-month response rate of 47%, with 28% remaining tumor free by 1 year. Furthermore, the response was modestly durable at 2 years with 21% remaining continuously disease free, which may have been augmented by the maintenance schedule of up to 10 monthly maintenance doses. Despite having what seemed to be a higher risk cohort than the Di Lorenzo randomized phase II trial, progression-free survival rates were improved with only 3 patients (5%) progressing to muscle-invasive bladder cancer. This trial remains the largest and most successful use of salvage gemcitabine in a cohort that most closely resembles a BCG unresponsive cohort as defined today—even so, their median time from last BCG treatment of approximately 7 months would make the majority of these BCG failures fall outside the 6-month window required by the modern definition of BCG unresponsive disease. Nevertheless, success in this trial has prompted more studies using gemcitabine in combination therapies and has solidified gemcitabine as a valuable agent in the salvage setting.

TAXANES

Docetaxel was the prototypical drug of the taxane class first pioneered in a phase I trial by McKiernan and colleagues[17] in 2006 at Columbia University. This phase I trial demonstrated an excellent safety profile and tolerability with only 10 of the 18 patients demonstrating grade 1 to 2 toxicity. Patients were treated with a dose escalation of 6 weekly instillations of docetaxel that reached the target dose of 75 mg in 100 mL. The cohort was composed of high-grade BCG-refractory bladder cancer failing a mean of 3 prior induction courses of intravesical therapy. With an initial impressive 3-month CR rate of 56% careful long-term follow-up study was warranted. After a median follow-up time of 4 years without maintenance therapy, a continued CR rate of 22% was observed.[18] Only 2 patients (11%) experienced progression to muscle invasion after 6 cystectomies (33%) were performed.

After encouraging results with salvage docetaxel, the same group also studied an enhanced taxane that used a nanoparticle albumin-bound delivery system in combination with paclitaxel (Abraxane).[19] The single arm phase II trial of 28 patients recruited patients with recurrent bladder cancer after at least one induction of BCG with or without IFN. Similar to the docetaxel study, the median number of intravesical therapies used before enrollment was 2 (range, 1–4), suggesting a majority of refractory disease. All but 1 patient could be considered high risk by today's definition because only 1 patient was treated for multifocal low-grade Ta pathology. Remarkably, all but 1 of the 10 initial complete responders (36%) at 6 weeks remained disease free at 1 year with 6 monthly maintenance treatments. Only 1 patient progressed to muscle-invasive bladder cancer after 9 patients (21%) had cystectomies. Longer term outcomes of this cohort showed an RFS of 18% at median follow-up of 41 months.[20] Notably, this population of patients were more heavily enriched with CIS (71%) versus the prior study of docetaxel that had 56% of patients with CIS at trial entry.[17] With comparable modest efficacy seen in both docetaxel/nab-paclitaxel and gemcitabine as salvage agents, it was only logical that these 2 agents be studied in combination for synergistic effect—a topic that will be thoroughly covered in Nathan A. Brooks and Michael A. O'Donnell's article, "Combination Intravesical Therapy," in this issue.

BACILLUS CALMETTE-GUÉRIN DERIVATIVES: MYCOBACTERIAL CELL WALL EXTRACT AND MYCOBACTERIAL CELL WALL NUCLEIC ACID COMPLEX

Not long after BCG was first successfully used in patients with bladder cancer, investigators began experimenting with compounds that they hoped would have a similar effect as BCG without the

risks involved in using a live attenuated bacterium. The first compound that showed promise was a mycobacterial cell wall extract (MCWE) from the nonpathogenic *Mycobacterium phlei* developed by Morales and colleagues[21] with initial studies in the early to mid-1990s focused on prostate cancer models in dogs and rats.[22] MCWE was first used in a mice bladder tumor model by Chin and colleagues,[23] who demonstrated significant tumor regression on MRI, prompting consideration for human use.

The first trial of MCWE in human bladder cancer was conducted by Morales and colleagues[24] in 2001 for patients with CIS. This was a single-arm trial of 61 patients of whom 46% received prior BCG induction. Patients underwent a 6-week induction course of a 4 mg MCWE oil emulsion reconstituted in 50 mL of saline followed by monthly maintenance dosing every month for 1 year. CR rates were 62% at 3 months and 41% at 1 year, although only 16 patients remained in the study by 1 year. The investigators noted fewer side effects than with the live BCG instillation and were surprised to find MCWE's efficacy to be similar between both BCG-naïve and BCG-exposed patients—this finding of efficacy after BCG spurred interest for study of this compound in the salvage setting. During experimentation with MCWE, investigators sought to strengthen its potency while lessening potential toxic side effects of MCWE, and the resulting related compound was called mycobacterial cell wall nucleic acid complex (MCNA). Like MCWE, MCNA is an immunomodulatory agent derived from mycobacterial cell wall fragments the nonpathogenic *M phlei* that are then activated with nucleic acids. It thus contains 5% to 10% of *M phlei* DNA, which is thought to mediate its therapeutic effect.[25] Ultimately, MCNA exerts its antitumor activity via both immunomodulation similar to BCG as well as having an added direct cytotoxic effect distinct from BCG.[25–27] Unlike MCWE that contained the potentially toxic mercury-based thimerosal, MCNA was isolated without the use of thimerosal and was thus deemed to have less potential toxicity.[28]

There are 2 substantial trials that have investigated the safety and efficacy of MCNA. In 2009, Morales and colleagues[28] published their dual arm trial comparing a 4 mg versus 8 mg dosing of MCNA in predominantly CIS patients. Eighty-five percent of the entire cohort had at least 1 prior BCG induction course and 35% had Ta/T1 disease that was fully resected before enrollment. After a 6-week induction of either 4 or 8 mg MCNA, patients were given 3-weekly maintenance dosing at 3 and 6 months. Response rates were modest with the immediate 3-month CR rates (defined as

Table 1
Summary of studies examining single agent salvage intravesical chemotherapy and BCG derivatives

First Author	Design	Patients	Treatment	Median Follow-Up	Recurrence-Free Survival	Prog. %	RC, %	Comments
Steinberg et al,[11] 2000	Single arm, phase I/II	n = 90, all ≥1 BCG induction, 70% with ≥2	Valrubicin 800 mg, 6 wk induction	30 mo	6 mo: 25% 1 y: 17% End of study: 8%	n/a	56%	Rate of progression not specified as suspected many owing to understaged TURs. 90% with local AEs, 3 unable to complete course.
Dinney et al,[12] 2013	Single modified arm, phase III	n = 80, all had ≥1 BCG induction, 39% with ≥2	Valrubicin 800 mg, 6 wk vs 9 wk	n/a	6 mo: 18% 1 y: 10% 2 y: 4%	n/a	25%	Most did not have progression; however, 4 patients died of bladder cancer.
Dalbagni et al,[14] 2006	Single arm, phase II	n = 30, BCG "refractory" or intolerant	Gemcitabine 2 g, × 12 biweekly doses over 7 wk	19 mo (0–35)	3 mo: 50% 1 y: 21%	7%	37%	Well-tolerated with only 36% patient developing local symptoms. No maintenance used.
Di Lorenzo et al,[15] 2010	RCT, gemcitabine vs second induction course of BCG	n = 80, all received 1 prior BCG, 30% LG	Gemcitabine 2 g biweekly ×6 weeks + maintenance vs BCG + maintenance ×3	15.5 mo (6–22)	Gem: 1 y, 55%; 2 y, 19% BCG: 1 y, 27%; 2 y (P<.008)	Gem: 33% BCG: 37.5%	Gem: 43% BCG: 40%	First and only RCT of gemcitabine vs BCG in this unique setting. High rates of disease progression and metastasis in both groups.
Skinner et al,[16] 2013	Single arm, phase II	n = 58, all received 2 prior BCG courses, 89% considered high risk	Gemcitabine 2 g/wk ×6 + monthly maintenance ×10	15 mo	3 mo: 47% 1 y: 28% 2 y: 21%	3.4%	26%	Only 3 patients had progression to MIBC at RC.

(continued on next page)

Table 1
(continued)

First Author	Design	Patients	Treatment	Median Follow-Up	Recurrence-Free Survival	Prog, %	RC, %	Comments
Laudano et al,[18] 2010	Single arm, phase I	n = 18, all had ≥1 BCG induction; mean of 3 prior IVT courses	Docetaxel escalating dose to 75 mg/100 mL NS ×6, no maintenance	4 y	1 y: 61% 2 y: 44% Median: 13.3 mo	11%	33%	4 (22%) patients remained disease free without further treatment.
McKiernan et al,[19] 2014	Single arm, phase II	n = 28, only 1 patient with low grade pathology, all received ≥1 prior BCG	Nab-paclitaxel, 500 mg/100 mL NS weekly ×6 + monthly maintenance ×6	21 mo (range, 5–47 mo)	3 mo: 36% 1 y: 36%	3%	32%	Median number of prior IVT was 2 with high enrichment of CIS (71%). Long-term follow-up of cohort showed RFS of 18% at median follow-up of 41 mo.[20]
Morales et al,[24] 2001	Single arm	n = 61, 46% prior BCG induction; all CIS	MCWE 6 wk induction + maintenance	Range, 3–12 mo; poor long-term follow-up	3 mo: 62.5%, 1 y: 41%	n/a	n/a	Similar rates of response in BCG-naïve patients and prior induction.
Morales et al,[28] 2009	Dual arm: 4 vs 8 mg MCNA	n = 55 85% prior BCG induction All with CIS, 35% also with Ta/T1 disease	MCNA 6 wk induction + maintenance	Range, 3–18 mo, median not given	4 mg: 3 mo, 40%, 1 y:40% 8 mg: 3 mo, 62%; 1 y, 33%	n/a	n/a	Similar adverse effects in both dosage groups (33%). 8 mg thought to be more effective.
Morales et al,[29] 2015	Single arm, phase III	n = 129, all received BCG, 82% BCG refractory	MCNA 8 mg, followed by 3 weekly maintenance ×5	34.7 mo	1 y: 25%, 2 y: 19% Papillary only tumors, 1-y RFS: 35%	22%	43%	21% of RC specimens had pT2 or greater, metastasis occurred in 10 (8%) patients.

Abbreviations: AE, adverse event; BCG, Bacillus Calmette-Guérin; CIS, carcinoma in situ; CR, complete response; IVT, intravesical therapy; MCNA, mycobacterial cell wall nucleic acid complex; MCWE, mycobacterial cell wall extract; MIBC, muscle-invasive bladder cancer; NMIBC, non-muscle-invasive bladder cancer; NS, normal saline; RC, radical cystectomy; RCT, randomized, controlled trial; RFS, recurrence-free survival; TUR, transurethral resection.

negative biopsy and cytology) between 40% (4 mg) to 62% (8 mg), with 1-year response rates fairly durable at 40% for the 4 mg group and 33% for the 8 mg group. Median follow-up was not given for this or the prior study, but there was clearly a large drop-out rate with only 11 of the 28 patients available for 12-month follow-up within the 8 mg group.

The largest phase III trial of MCNA was conducted across 25 sites in North America from 2006 to 2011 by Morales and colleagues.[29] It was a single-arm trial of 129 patients treated with a 6 weekly induction course of 8 mg MCNA followed by 3 weekly maintenance induction cycles for 2 years that resembled the SWOG protocol (at months 3, 6, 12, 18, and 24). The population was predominantly high grade with CIS, with only 7.8% of patients having low grade Ta pathology and 29.5% having only papillary tumors. All patients had prior exposure to BCG with 83% of patients relapsing within 1 year of BCG treatment with the remaining patients relapsing after prolonged disease-free periods. Patients received a mean of 12 MCNA instillations with 99% compliance rate for planned instillations—only 2 patients discontinued treatment owing to adverse effects. Median follow-up of the entire cohort was much improved from the prior MCWE/MCNA studies at 34.7 months. A total of 30 patients were considered responders for an overall 1-year RFS rate of 25% (median RFS, 5.7 months). Notably, patients who were disease free at 1-year were likely to have a durable response as only 4 of 30 patients (13%) of these patients eventually recurred and required cystectomy. Overall Progression rates were fairly high however, with (22%) of patients experiencing progression, of which 11 had localized muscle-invasive bladder cancer, 10 progressed with metastasis, and 7 died from bladder cancer. A total of 43% of these patients ultimately underwent cystectomy, of whom 21% had pT2 disease or greater.

Although these results do not appear particularly impressive, historical CR rates for salvage regimens in patients who are truly BCG unresponsive (BCG refractory + relapsing), rarely exceed RFS rates of more than 20% at 1 year. Indeed, valrubicin, the only FDA-approved intravesical therapy for CIS failing BCG, had only an 18% CR rate at 6 months in patients with CIS who would be considered BCG failures by today's definition.[11] In comparison, this MCNA study found the overall CR rate of 34% at 6 months in patients with CIS failing prior BCG.

Overall, MCNA is likely comparable to other single agent salvage intravesical therapies for BCG failure. Moreover, MCNA has been shown to have lower toxicity compared with BCG, especially in regards to systemic adverse events, with reported side effects that may be comparable with an intravesical chemotherapy such as gemcitabine. Despite these modestly encouraging results, there seems to be little interest in further developing mechanisms to enhance the efficacy of this modality, and intravesical BCG derivative therapy is not currently commercially available. With a production process distinct from BCG's in using a different mycobacterium from the *Mycobacterium bovis* used in production of BCG, the ongoing shortages of BCG may spark renewed interest in therapies with cell wall complexes in both BCG naïve and BCG unresponsive setting.

REFERENCES

1. Kamat AM, Sylvester RJ, Bohle A, et al. Definitions, end points, and clinical trial designs for non-muscle-invasive bladder cancer: recommendations from the International Bladder Cancer Group. J Clin Oncol 2016;34(16):1935–44.
2. Solsona E, Iborra I, Dumont R, et al. The 3-month clinical response to intravesical therapy as a predictive factor for progression in patients with high risk superficial bladder cancer. J Urol 2000;164(3 Pt 1): 685–9.
3. Gallagher BL, Joudi FN, Maymi JL, et al. Impact of previous Bacille Calmette-Guerin failure pattern on subsequent response to Bacille Calmette-Guerin plus interferon intravesical therapy. Urology 2008; 71(2):297–301.
4. Chang SS, Boorjian SA, Chou R, et al. Diagnosis and treatment of non-muscle invasive bladder cancer: AUA/SUO guideline. J Urol 2016;196(4):1021–9.
5. Paz MM, Zhang X, Lu J, et al. A new mechanism of action for the anticancer drug mitomycin C: mechanism-based inhibition of thioredoxin reductase. Chem Res Toxicol 2012;25(7):1502–11.
6. Bohle A, Jocham D, Bock PR. Intravesical bacillus Calmette-Guerin versus mitomycin C for superficial bladder cancer: a formal meta-analysis of comparative studies on recurrence and toxicity. J Urol 2003; 169(1):90–5.
7. Shelley MD, Wilt TJ, Court J, et al. Intravesical bacillus Calmette-Guerin is superior to mitomycin C in reducing tumour recurrence in high-risk superficial bladder cancer: a meta-analysis of randomized trials. BJU Int 2004;93(4):485–90.
8. Malmstrom PU, Sylvester RJ, Crawford DE, et al. An individual patient data meta-analysis of the long-term outcome of randomised studies comparing intravesical mitomycin C versus bacillus Calmette-Guerin for non-muscle-invasive bladder cancer. Eur Urol 2009;56(2):247–56.

9. Babjuk M, Bohle A, Burger M, et al. EAU guidelines on non-muscle-invasive urothelial carcinoma of the bladder: update 2016. Eur Urol 2017;71(3):447–61.

10. Minotti G, Menna P, Salvatorelli E, et al. Anthracyclines: molecular advances and pharmacologic developments in antitumor activity and cardiotoxicity. Pharmacol Rev 2004;56(2):185–229.

11. Steinberg G, Bahnson R, Brosman S, et al. Efficacy and safety of valrubicin for the treatment of Bacillus Calmette-Guerin refractory carcinoma in situ of the bladder. The Valrubicin Study Group. J Urol 2000; 163(3):761–7.

12. Dinney CP, Greenberg RE, Steinberg GD. Intravesical valrubicin in patients with bladder carcinoma in situ and contraindication to or failure after bacillus Calmette-Guerin. Urol Oncol 2013;31(8):1635–42.

13. Messing EM, Tangen CM, Lerner SP, et al. Effect of intravesical instillation of gemcitabine vs saline immediately following resection of suspected low-grade non-muscle-invasive bladder cancer on tumor recurrence: SWOG S0337 randomized clinical trial. JAMA 2018;319(18):1880–8.

14. Dalbagni G, Russo P, Bochner B, et al. Phase II trial of intravesical gemcitabine in Bacille Calmette-Guerin-refractory transitional cell carcinoma of the bladder. J Clin Oncol 2006;24(18):2729–34.

15. Di Lorenzo G, Perdona S, Damiano R, et al. Gemcitabine versus Bacille Calmette-Guerin after initial Bacille Calmette-Guerin failure in non-muscle-invasive bladder cancer: a multicenter prospective randomized trial. Cancer 2010;116(8):1893–900.

16. Skinner EC, Goldman B, Sakr WA, et al. SWOG S0353: phase II trial of intravesical gemcitabine in patients with nonmuscle invasive bladder cancer and recurrence after 2 prior courses of intravesical bacillus Calmette-Guerin. J Urol 2013;190(4): 1200–4.

17. McKiernan JM, Masson P, Murphy AM, et al. Phase I trial of intravesical docetaxel in the management of superficial bladder cancer refractory to standard intravesical therapy. J Clin Oncol 2006;24(19): 3075–80.

18. Laudano MA, Barlow LJ, Murphy AM, et al. Long-term clinical outcomes of a phase I trial of intravesical docetaxel in the management of non-muscle-invasive bladder cancer refractory to standard intravesical therapy. Urology 2010;75(1):134–7.

19. McKiernan JM, Holder DD, Ghandour RA, et al. Phase II trial of intravesical nanoparticle albumin bound paclitaxel for the treatment of nonmuscle invasive urothelial carcinoma of the bladder after bacillus Calmette-Guerin treatment failure. J Urol 2014; 192(6):1633–8.

20. Robins DJ, Sui W, Matulay JT, et al. Long-term survival outcomes with intravesical nanoparticle albumin-bound paclitaxel for recurrent non-muscle-invasive bladder cancer after previous bacillus Calmette-Guerin Therapy. Urology 2017;103: 149–53.

21. Morales A, Nickel JC, Manley PN. Induction of controlled prostatic tissue necrosis by Bacille Calmette-Guerin derivatives. Urol Res 1991;19(1): 35–8.

22. Morales A, Nickel JC, Downey J, et al. Immunotherapy of an experimental adenocarcinoma of the prostate. J Urol 1995;153(5):1706–10.

23. Chin JL, Kadhim SA, Batislam E, et al. Mycobacterium cell wall: an alternative to intravesical bacillus Calmette Guerin (BCG) therapy in orthotopic murine bladder cancer. J Urol 1996;156(3): 1189–93.

24. Morales A, Chin JL, Ramsey EW. Mycobacterial cell wall extract for treatment of carcinoma in situ of the bladder. J Urol 2001;166(5):1633–7 [discussion: 1637–8].

25. Filion MC, Phillips NC. Therapeutic potential of mycobacterial cell wall-DNA complexes. Expert Opin Investig Drugs 2001;10(12):2157–65.

26. Filion MC, Lepicier P, Morales A, et al. Mycobacterium phlei cell wall complex directly induces apoptosis in human bladder cancer cells. Br J Cancer 1999;79(2):229–35.

27. Filion MC, Filion B, Reader S, et al. Modulation of interleukin-12 synthesis by DNA lacking the CpG motif and present in a mycobacterial cell wall complex. Cancer Immunol Immunother 2000;49(6): 325–34.

28. Morales A, Phadke K, Steinhoff G. Intravesical mycobacterial cell wall-DNA complex in the treatment of carcinoma in situ of the bladder after standard intravesical therapy has failed. J Urol 2009; 181(3):1040–5.

29. Morales A, Herr H, Steinberg G, et al. Efficacy and safety of MCNA in patients with nonmuscle invasive bladder cancer at high risk for recurrence and progression after failed treatment with bacillus Calmette-Guerin. J Urol 2015;193(4):1135–43.

Heated Intravesical Chemotherapy
Biology and Clinical Utility

Wei Phin Tan, MD, Thomas A. Longo, MD, Brant A. Inman, MD, MS*

KEYWORDS

• Bladder hyperthermia • Heated chemotherapy • Heated mitomycin • Intravesical chemotherapy
• Intravesical mitomycin • HIVEC

KEY POINTS

• Heat can improve drug delivery, increase cancer cell sensitivity to therapeutic agents, and trigger anticancer immune responses.
• Three methods of bladder heating are available clinically: external deep regional radiofrequency heating, intravesical catheter radiofrequency heating, and recirculating conductive heating.
• Administering intravesical chemotherapy with heat is safe and seems to improve treatment efficacy.

INTRODUCTION

Bladder cancer (BC) is the fourth most commonly diagnosed cancer in men and more than 75% are non–muscle invasive BC (NMIBC) at diagnosis.[1,2] NMIBC is generally treated with transurethral resection of the bladder tumor (TURBT) as a first step. In high-grade tumors, a repeat TURBT is often performed to ensure complete tumor removal and the absence of muscle-invasive cancer.[3] Patients determined—based on grade, stage, number of tumors, size of tumors, and so on—to be at intermediate or high risk of recurrence are usually treated with adjuvant intravesical chemotherapy or Bacillus Calmette-Guerin (BCG). BCG-treated patients are generally offered maintenance therapy for 1 year if they fall under intermediate risk or 3 years if they are high risk.[4] Despite these years of active therapy, many (up to one-half) patients with NMIBC experience a disease recurrence.[5] For those patients whose tumors are BCG unresponsive, radical cystectomy is the standard of care salvage treatment, but carries a significant morbidity and mortality risk.[6] For this reason, most patients faced with the prospect of cystectomy inquire about bladder preserving alternatives and one such alternative is the combination of intravesical chemotherapy with heat.

HYPERTHERMIA AS A TREATMENT FOR NON–MUSCLE-INVASIVE BLADDER CANCER

The application of mild fever range heat (40°C–44°C) to the bladder is called hyperthermia (HT).[7] HT is different from thermal ablation where temperatures reach 60°C to 90°C. In general, HT can be used to (1) improve drug delivery to the bladder, (2) kill malignant urothelial cells directly, (3) improve BC sensitivity to chemotherapy, and (4) trigger anticancer immune responses.[8–10]

Disclosures: Dr W.P. Tan is supported by the Ruth L. Kirschstein NRSA Institutional Research Training Grant (T32-CA093245). Dr B.A. Inman has received clinical trial or research support from the following entities within the past 12 months: Abbott Laboratories, Bristol-Myers Squibb, Urogen, Anchiano Therapeutics, Nucleix, Taris Biomedical, Combat Medical, FKD Therapies, Dendreon, and Genentech. He has consulted for ColdGenesys.
Division of Urology, Duke University Medical Center, Durham, NC 27710, USA
* Corresponding author. Box 103868, 3007 Snyderman Building, 905 La Salle Street, Durham, NC 27710.
E-mail address: brant.inman@duke.edu

Drug Delivery

When a tumor is heated to between 38°C to 42°C, several important vascular physiologic effects occur. Local vasodilation occurs and results in increased blood flow to the tumor and adjacent tissue.[11] The warmer environment causes the lipid–protein membrane bilayer that contains cells to become more permeable, resulting in easier drug penetration into the cell through the cell membrane. These 2 mechanisms work synergistically to make an already leaky tumor vasculature even leakier, a phenomenon known as the enhanced permeability and retention effect.[12] By increasing the enhanced permeability and retention effect, HT improves drug delivery to bladder tumors, which in turn leads to better tumor cell destruction.

Cytotoxicity

Because tumors are characterized by a constant state of a relatively inadequate resource supply, their microenvironment develops a hypoxic, acidotic, and energy-deprived character.[13] HT to greater than 42°C further alters blood flow to the tumor microenvironment, further depriving the tumor of the oxygen and nutrients that it needs to survive.[13] Morphologic changes observed when this occurs include an outflow of cytoplasm into the interstitial space, endothelial swelling, changes of the viscosity of blood cell membranes, and microthrombosis.[11,14] Tumor cells are more sensitive to HT than normal urothelial cells and therefore suffer a lot more during mild heating.

Improving Sensitivity to Therapeutic Agents

Multiple antineoplastic agents have been shown to be more efficacious when administered to a heated tumor,[11] and the thermal enhancement ratio (TER) quantifies the degree to which heat affects drug efficacy.[15] The TER compares the ratio of cell kill at 43°C to that at 37°C, with drugs possessing a TER of greater than 1 working better with heat. Chemotherapeutic agents used to treat BC such as cisplatin, mitomycin C (MMC), gemcitabine, and doxorubicin all have a TER of greater than 1.3.[16] It is noteworthy that the timing of heating relative to chemotherapy exposure may be important. For example, gemcitabine seems to work better when administered 24 hours after HT.[17]

Anticancer Immune Responses

Temperature is a well-known regulator of immune function.[18] Some relevant effects of HT on immunity include changes in number and phenotype of tumor-infiltrating leukocytes, improved tumor-infiltrating leukocyte function, and cytokine release.[19] HT also causes heat shock protein release from tumor cells, particularly heat shock protein 70 and heat shock protein 90, resulting in the cross-priming of antigen-specific cytotoxic T lymphocytes.[20] The consequence is that HT-treated tumors actively participate in their own demise by leading to a form of self-vaccination.

METHODS OF DELIVERING BLADDER HYPERTHERMIA

Although there are many ways to categorize devices for HT, the most obvious category to both the patient and the clinician is how the heat is delivered, namely, external vs internal. External devices use energy emitters to apply heat to a field within the body. They incorporate treatment planning systems to optimize the dose delivered and minimize damage to adjacent tissue, similar to the dose planning used in radiation therapy.

External Devices

One type of external heating is deep regional radiofrequency, which uses an array of radiofrequency emitters to focus heat into the body. These devices require a medical physics team and a radiofrequency shielded room, which increases cost and decreases generalizability to office-based locations where NMIBC is typically treated. Furthermore, owing to the risk of heating implanted metal, external radiofrequency-based heating is generally contraindicated in patients with implanted medical devices (eg, pacemakers) and hip replacements.[21] The BSD 2000 system (Pyresar Medical, Salt Lake City UT) is an example of an external deep regional radiofrequency device. It uses electromagnetic phased array applicators to deliver deep tissue HT and allows control of the 3-dimensional pattern of therapy specific to the patient's tumor.[22–26] For bladder HT, the patient has temperature probes placed in the rectum and bladder to monitor the internal temperature. A water-filled applicator is then placed over the lower abdomen/pelvis and water is circulated to cool the skin during therapy. Another example is the AMC device, now sold as the Alba 4D system (Medlogix, Rome, Italy), which also uses radiofrequency arrayed systems to achieve deep tissue HT.[22,27–29] As with the BSD system, it is coupled with a water bolus temperature control apparatus. Other electromagnetic systems include the Thermotron, CanCure, Dubai, UAE (only available in North Africa and the Middle East) and the Celsius42 devices (Celsisus42, Eschweiler, Germany). A significant advantage of the Celsius42 system is that it does not require a shielded room, although its use has not been studied in NMIBC.

High-intensity focused ultrasound (HIFU) is another form of external heating. As the name suggests, HIFU uses the focused soundwaves in an accurate and specific manner to increase the temperature of the tumor without harming adjacent tissue. The commercially available HIFU systems are large devices that externally deliver HIFU. There is a laparoscopic probe that uses a single transducer to image and deliver HIFU to the tumor in a more precise, albeit invasive manner.[30]

Internal Devices

Internal devices lack the depth of penetration of external devices but have the significant advantage of delivering heat almost exclusively to the bladder. There are 2 systems that use conductive HT the Combat bladder recirculating system (BRS) (innoMedicus, Cham, Switzerland) and Unithermia (ElMedical, Hod-Hasharon, Israel).[31,32] Both devices externally heat fluid and the circulate it to the bladder via a 3-way irrigating Foley catheter. The recirculating fluid contains a chemotherapy agent chosen by the treating physician. Recirculating systems are the smallest, most portable, and least expensive bladder heaters. Synergo (Tigard, OR) produces a third intravesical bladder heating system that also uses recirculating bladder irrigation, but instead of a heat exchanger it uses a microwave radiofrequency emitting intravesical catheter to heat the bladder.[33–35] The Synergo device is presently the most well-studied device among those mentioned, although several large trials of the Combat BRS device have accrued and will report results soon.

There are 2 additional devices worth mentioning, electromotive drug administration (EMDA) and nanoparticles. Although in the strict sense, these are not HT devices, they do share a similar therapeutic mechanism. EMDA uses a urethral catheter to deliver ionized drugs intravesically. Dispersive pads (similar to electrocautery) are placed on the lower abdomen and an electric current is applied intravesically to drive the drug into the urothelium at a rate proportional to the amount of current being applied. EMDA allows for greater depth of penetration than would be achievable by passive diffusion alone.[36] Nanoparticles can be administered intravenously or intravesically and they preferentially accumulate in tumors secondary to the enhanced permeability and retention effect.[37] Externally delivered light or alternating magnetic fields generates heat in the tissue hosting the nanoparticles.

CLINICAL EXPERIENCE WITH BLADDER HYPERTHERMIA

The combination of heat and intravesical chemotherapy has been used both in the neoadjuvant (before TURBT) and adjuvant settings (after TURBT). For this review, we use HIVEC as the acronym for hyperthermic intravesical chemotherapy. The large majority of HIVEC treatments done thus far have used MMC as the chemotherapy agent.

Phase I and II Trials

To date, there are 5 clinical trials of neoadjuvant chemo ablative HIVEC for NMIBC and all used MMC. In these trials, 60% to 100% of patients had previously undergone some form of intravesical therapy (**Table 1**). The complete response rate of patients who underwent HIVEC ranged from 53% to 75% with a partial response rate of 20% to 47%. The recurrence rate ranged from 13% to 39% at a median follow-up of 15 to 39 months.[34,38–41]

The first trial of MMC HIVEC was conducted by Colombo and colleagues[39] in 1995, where 44 patients underwent neoadjuvant administration of intravesical chemotherapy and simultaneous local bladder HT for eight 60-minute sessions done twice weekly, followed by TURBT 3 weeks later. The complete response rate was 70%, partial response was 20% and no response in 9% of patients. After a mean follow-up of 24 months, 16% recurred.[39] In 2004, Gofrit and colleagues[34] treated 52 patients with high-grade NMIBC with MMC HIVEC. Of these, 28 men were treated with neoadjuvant HIVEC (MMC 80 mg) and 24 men adjuvant HIVEC (MMC 40 mg). More than 50% of both groups have been previously treated with BCG. Recurrence-free survival was 71% at a median follow-up of 15 months. Surprisingly, in the neoadjuvant cohort, 75% of patients achieved complete response to therapy.[34] Subsequently, there were 2 randomized trials conducted by Colombo and colleagues[40,41] where neoadjuvant HIVEC (MMC 40 mg) was compared with standard MMC, or to EMDA (MMC 40 mg) and standard MMC. HIVEC achieved a complete response in 66% of patients in both studies, compared with 22% for standard MMC and 40% for EMDA.[40,41]

There are 3 phase I and II adjuvant trials reporting recurrence-free survival. In these 3 trials, the patient cohort consisted of intermediate and high-grade NMIBC. The 1- and 2-year recurrence-free survival rates range from 67% to 87% and 50% to 91%, respectively (**Table 2**). Soria and colleagues[32] used the Unithermia device, which delivers heat via conducting heating. In

Table 1
Phase I and II trials and observational studies on neoadjuvant intravesical chemothermia therapy

Author and Year	Study Design	Sample Size	Treatment	Heat Source	Induction Schedule	Maintenance Schedule for CR Group	Patients with Previous Intravesical Treatment (%)	Follow-up	CR (%)	PR (%)	NR (%)	Recurrence Rate (%)
Colombo et al,[39] 1995	Phase I	44	30 mg MMC in 60 mL water for 40 min	Synergo (42.5–44.5°C)	Twice weekly within 6 wk (total of 8 sessions)	—	63.6	24 mo (mean)	70.4	20.4	9.1	15.9
Gofrit et al,[34] 2004	Phase I	28	(40 mg MMC dissolved in 50 mL of distilled water for 20 min) ×2	Synergo (42 ± 2°C)	Once weekly ×8	Once monthly ×4	60.1	15.2 mo	75	—	—	19
Sousa et al,[38] 2014	Phase I	15	80 mg MMC dissolved in 50 mL of distilled water for 60 min	Combat BRS (42 ± 1°C)	Once weekly ×8	Partial responder treated once weekly ×4, then once monthly ×11. CR did not received maintenance	74	29 mo	53	47	0	13.3
Colombo et al,[40] 1996	Phase II	29	(40 mg MMC in 50 mL distilled water for 30 min) ×2	Synergo (42.5–46°C for 60 min)	Once/twice weekly ×6–8	—	100	38 mo	66	34	0	27
		23	40 mg MMC in 50 mL sterile water for 60 min	—	Once/twice-weekly ×6–8	—	100	36 mo	22	26	52	39

Reference	Study type	No. of patients	MMC regimen	Device (temperature)	Schedule			Follow-up				
Colombo,[41] 2001	Phase II	36	40 mg MMC in 50 mL of saline for 60 min	—	Once weekly ×4	—		—	27.7	—	—	
		29	40 mg MMC diluted in 50 mL of distilled water for 60 min	Synergo (mean of 42.5°C)	Once weekly ×4	—		—	66	—	—	
		15	40 mg MMC dissolved in 150 mL of distilled water and EMDA for 20 min	Physionizer 30	Once weekly ×4	—		—	40	—	—	
Rigatti et al,[35] 1991	Observational	12	30 mg MMC dissolved in 60 mL of distilled water for 60 min	SB-TS 100 (41.5–43.5°C)	Once/twice-weekly ×6–8	—		16 mo	41.7	33.3	25	8.3
Moskovitz et al,[48] 2005	Observational	10	(40 mg MMC dissolved in 50 mL of distilled water for 30 min) ×2	Synergo (42 ± 2°C)	Once weekly ×8	Once monthly ×4	80	5.6 mo (mean)	80	—	—	
Witjes,[49] 2009	Observational	26 (100% CIS)	(40 mg MMC dissolved in 50 mL of distilled water for 30 min) ×2	Synergo (41–44°C) for 60 min	Once weekly ×6	Once every 6 wk ×6 (total of 6 sessions)	66.7	22 mo	92	—	—	22

(continued on next page)

Table 1
(continued)

Author and Year	Study Design	Sample Size	Treatment	Heat Source	Induction Schedule	Maintenance Schedule for CR Group	Patients with Previous Intravesical Treatment (%)	Follow-up	CR (%)	PR (%)	NR (%)	Recurrence Rate (%)
Moskovitz et al,[50] 2012	Observational	26	(40 mg MMC dissolved in 50 mL of distilled water for 30 min) ×2	Synergo (approximately 42°C)	Once weekly ×8	Once every 6 wk for first year (20 mg MMC)	76.9	9 mo	79	8	13	16
Volpe et al,[51] 2012	Observational	14	(40 mg MMC dissolved in 50 mL of distilled water for 30 min) ×2	Synergo (42 ± 2°C)	Once weekly ×8	Once monthly ×6	100	14 mo (mean)	42.9	9.9	47.2	46.3
Sousa et al,[31] 2016	Observational	24	80 mg MMC dissolved in 50 mL of distilled water for 60 min	Combat (43 ± 0.5°C)	Once weekly ×8	Once monthly ×6	33	37 mo	62.5	33.3	4.2	31.3

Dose in the maintenance group is similar to treatment unless stated otherwise.
Abbreviations: BRS, bladder recirculating system; CIS, carcinoma in situ; CR, complete response; HT, hyperthermia therapy; NR, no response; PR, partial response.

Table 2
Phase I, II, and III trials and observational studies on adjuvant intravesical chemothermia therapy

Author and Year Published	Trial	Sample Size	Treatment per Session	Heat Source	Induction Schedule	Maintenance Schedule for CR Group	Risk Group (% Patients)	Hx of Intravesical Therapy (% Patients)	Follow-up, Median (IQR)	1-y RFS (%)	2-y RFS (%)	5-y RFS (%)
Gofrit et al,[34] 2004	Phase I	24	(20 mg MMC in 50 mL of distilled water for 20 min) ×2	Synergo (42 ± 2°C)	Once weekly ×8	Once monthly ×4	High grade (100)	87.5	35.3 mo (mean)	66.5	60.6	52.1
Soria et al,[32] 2016	Phase I and 2	34	(40 mg MMC in 50 mL saline for 22 min) ×2	Unithermia (42.5 ± 1°C)	Once weekly ×6	Once monthly ×4	High grade (53) Low grade (47)	100	41 (–)	85.4	73.5	55.2
van der Heijden et al,[42] 2004	Phase II	90	(20 mg MMC in 50 mL of distilled water for 30/60 min) ×2/1	Synergo (41–44°C)	Once weekly ×6–8	Once monthly ×4–6	High risk (41) Intermediate risk (59)	66.1	18 (4–24)	86.7	75.4	—
Colombo et al,[43] 2003	Phase III	42	(20 mg MMC in 50 mL of distilled water for 30 min) ×2	Synergo (42 ± 2°C)	Once weekly ×8	Once monthly ×4	High grade (90.5)	—	24 mo (–)	88.7	82.8	61.7
		41	20 mg MMC in 50 mL of distilled water for 60 min	—	Once weekly ×8	Once monthly ×4	High grade (97.6)	—		50.3	38.4	21.3
Arends et al,[44] 2016	Phase III	92	(20 mg MMC in 50 mL of distilled water for 30 min) ×2	Synergo (42 ± 2°C)	Once weekly ×6	Once every 6 wk for the first year	High grade (81.6) Low grade (18.4)	52	24 mo (–)	90.5	80.2	—
		98	BCG (Oncotice) full dose for 120 min	—	Once weekly ×6	Three weekly doses at 3, 6, and 12 mo	Intermediate risk (67.4 High risk (32.6	—		75.8	66.5	—

(continued on next page)

Table 2
(continued)

Author and Year Published	Trial	Sample Size	Treatment per Session	Heat Source	Induction Schedule	Maintenance Schedule for CR Group	Risk Group (% Patients)	Hx of Intravesical Therapy (% Patients)	Follow-up, Median (IQR)	1-y RFS (%)	2-y RFS (%)	5-y RFS (%)
Tan et al,[45] 2019	Phase III	48	(20 mg MMC in 50 mL of distilled water for 30 min) ×2	Synergo (42 ± 2°C)	Once weekly ×6	Once every 6 wk for the first year, once every 8 wk for the second year	High grade (100)	100	36 mo (range, 23.1–44.5 mo)	49.8	35	—
		56	BCG or standard of care at institution	—	Once weekly ×6	Three weekly instillations at 3, 6, 12, 18, and 24 mo	High grade (100)	100		56.7	42.1	—
Moskovitz et al,[48] 2005	Observational	22	(20 mg MMC dissolved in 50 mL of distilled water for 30 min) ×2	Synergo (42 ± 2°C)	Once weekly ×6–8	Once monthly ×4–6	High grade (68.2) Low grade (31.8)	63.5	9.6 mo (mean)	100	70	—
Nativ et al,[52] 2009	Observational	111	(20 mg MMC in 50 mL solution for 30 min) ×2	Synergo (42 ± 2°C)	Once weekly ×6	Once every 4–6 wk ×6	High grade (61) Low grade (39)	100	16 mo (range, 2–74 mo)	85	56	—
Halachmi et al,[53] 2011	Observational	56	(20 mg MMC for 30 min) ×2	Synergo (42 ± 2°C)	Once weekly ×6	Once every 4–6 wk ×6	High grade (100)	54	18 mo (range, 2–49 mo)	77	42.9	—
Moskovitz et al,[50] 2012	Observational	66	(20 mg MMC in 50 mL solution for 30 min) ×2	Synergo (approximately 42°C)	Once weekly ×6	Once every 6 wk for first year	High grade (45.5) Low grade (51.5) Not reported (1.5)	74.2	23 mo (range, 3–84 mo)	86.5	67.2	—
Volpe et al,[51] 2012	Observational	16	(20 mg MMC dissolved in 50 mL of distilled water for 30 min) ×2	Synergo (42 ± 2°C)	Once weekly ×6	Once monthly ×6	High grade (100)	100	14 mo (mean)	87.5	58.6	—

Study	Design	N	Dose	HT device	Induction	Maintenance	Grade/Risk		Follow-up			
Maffezzini et al,[54] 2014	Observational	42	40 mg MMC dissolved in 50 mL of distilled water for 60 min	Synergo (42.5 ± 1.5°C)	Once weekly ×4	Once every 2 wk ×6, then once monthly ×4	High grade (100)	64.3	38 mo (range, 4–73 mo)	88.1	80.2	63.5
Ekin et al,[55] 2015 (APJCP)	Observational	43	40 mg MMC dissolved in 50 mL of distilled water for 60 min	UniThermia (42.5–45°C)	Once weekly ×6	Three weekly instillations at month 3 and 6	High grade (58.1) Low grade (41.9)	—	30 mo (range, 9–39 mo)	82	61	—
Ekin et al,[56] 2015 (CJU)	Observational	40	40 mg MMC in 50 mL saline solution for 60 min	UniThermia (42.5–45°C)	Once weekly ×6	Three-weekly instillations at month 3 and 6	High grade (60) Low grade (40)	—	33 mo (range, 24–39 mo)	92.2	73.6	—
Sooriakumaran et al,[57] 2016	Observational	97	40 mg MMC dissolved in 50 mL of normal saline for 60 min	Synergo (41–44°C)	Once weekly ×6–8	Once every 6 wk for the first year, one every 8 wk for the second year (20 mg MMC)	High grade (100)	90.7	27 mo (range, 16–47 mo)	82.7	66.0	48.6
Sousa et al,[32] 2016	Observational	16	40 mg MMC dissolved in 50 mL of distilled water for 60 min	Combat (43 ± 0.5°C)	Once weekly ×4	No	High risk (71) Intermediate risk (29)	81.3	24 mo	100	88.1	—

Dose in the maintenance group is similar to treatment unless stated otherwise.

Abbreviations: BCG, Bacillus Calmette-Guerin; CR, complete response; HT, hyperthermia therapy; Hx, history; IQR, interquartile range; RFS, recurrence free survival.

this study, 34 patients with recurrent, intermediate risk NMIBC underwent a 6-week course of HIVEC (MMC 40 mg) for 45 minutes. The 1-, 2-, and 5-year RFS were 85%, 74%, and 55%, respectively. The other 2 trials used the Synergo system in high- and intermediate-risk NMIBC. Patients in both studies received 2 30-minute sessions of HIVEC (MMC 20 mg) for 6 to 8 cycles. The 1- and 2-year RFS ranged from 67% to 87% and 61% to 75%.[34,42]

Phase III Trials

To date, there are no phase III trials using neoadjuvant HIVEC for NMIBC, but there are 3 adjuvant HIVEC trials. In 2003, Colombo and colleagues[43] randomized 83 patients (>50% with high risk NMIBC) to HIVEC versus standard MMC. In both arms, patients received 20 mg/50 mL of MMC for two 30-minute sessions for 6 weeks. The 2-year RFS and 5-year RFS were 83% versus 38% and 62% versus 21% for HIVEC and standard MMC, respectively. The hazard ratio for HIVEC was 0.21.

Arends and colleagues[44] subsequently reported a phase III randomized, controlled trial where 190 patients with intermediate and high risk NMIBC were randomized to HIVEC or BCG. Patients in the BCG arm received induction OncoTICE BCG + maintenance at 3, 6, and 12 months. HIVEC patients received MMC (20 mg/50 mL) for 2 30-minute sessions for 6 weeks, and maintenance course (3 cycles) at 3, 6, and 12 months. The 2-year RFS was better for HIVEC (82%) than BCG (65%).

More recently, in the HYMN trial 104 patients with BCG unresponsive NMIBC were randomized to HIVEC (MMC 20 mg/50 mL) versus standard MMC. Patients received induction followed by 3 once-weekly maintenance instillations at 3, 6, 12, 18, and 24 months. There was no statistical difference in RFS between the arms at 2 years (hazard ratio, 1.33; 95% confidence interval, 0.84–2.10; $P = .23$).[45] At a median follow-up of 35 months, the rate of disease progression was 8%.

In addition to the trials noted, there are 6 observational studies of neoadjuvant HIVEC and 10 of adjuvant HIVEC and these are summarized in **Tables 1** and **2**.[28,31,35,46–57] Recurrence-free survival curves from the various studies using the Synergo, Combat BRS and Unithermia devices are pooled and shown in **Fig. 1**.

CLINICAL EXPERIENCE WITH ELECTROMOTIVE DRUG ADMINISTRATION

The combination of MMC and EMDA has been used both in the neoadjuvant (before TURBT)

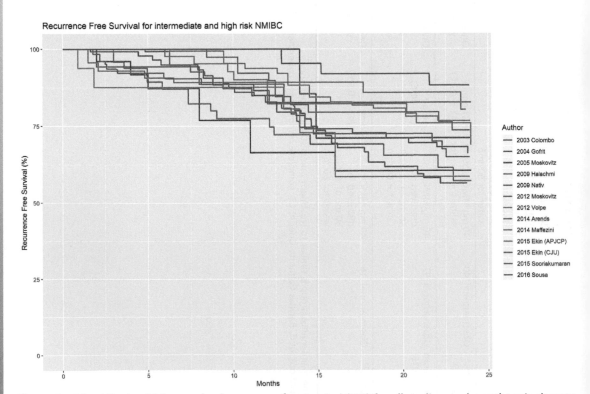

Fig. 1. Combined Kaplan-Meier graph of recurrence free survival (RFS) for all studies on chemothermia therapy for intermediate and high risk non-muscle invasive bladder cancer.

Table 3
Adverse events from Phase I, II, and III trials and observational studies on intravesical chemothermia

Author, Year	Study Type	N	Energy	Complete Treatment (%)	Grade ≥3 Adverse Events (%)	Hematuria (%)	UTI or Sepsis (%)	Stricture (%)	Allergic Reaction (%)
Colombo et al,[39] 1995	Phase I	44	RITE	—	—	—	—	2	2
Gofrit et al,[34] 2004	Phase I	52	RITE	96	—	2	10	2	10
Sousa et al,[38] 2014	Phase I	15	Conduction	—	0	20	13	0	7
Soria et al,[32] 2016	Phase I/II	34	Conduction	88	12	—	4	—	—
Colombo et al,[40] 1996	Phase II	29	RITE	93	—	—	—	0	—
Colombo et al,[41] 2001	Phase II	29	RITE	100	0	—	—	—	—
van der Heijden et al,[42] 2004	Phase II	90	RITE	100	—	9	0	4	9
Colombo et al,[43] 2003	Phase III	42	RITE	69	—	7	0	7	12
Arends et al,[44] 2016	Phase III	184	RITE	—	—	—	—	—	—
Tan and Kelly,[65] 2018	Phase III	48	RITE	90	10	48	23	6	15
Moskovitz et al,[48] 2005	Observational	47	RITE	—	4	17	0	6	4
Nativ et al,[52] 2009	Observational	111	RITE	95	8	19	2	5	8

(continued on next page)

Table 3
(continued)

Author, Year	Study Type	N	Energy	Complete Treatment (%)	Grade ≥3 Adverse Events (%)	Hematuria (%)	UTI or Sepsis (%)	Stricture (%)	Allergic Reaction (%)
Alfred Witjes et al,[49] 2009	Observational	26	RITE	92	—	3%	—	—	—
Halachmi et al,[67] 2011	Observational	56	RITE	91	—	4	0	2	12.5
Moskovitz et al,[50] 2012	Observational	92	RITE	96	4	7	1	5	1
Volpe et al,[51] 2012	Observational	30	RITE	100	—	27	7	0	13
Maffezzini et al,[54] 2014	Observational	42	RITE	88	0	62	0	0	0
Ekin et al,[55] 2015 (APJCP)	Observational	43	Conductive	93	12	9	0	0	7
Ekin et al,[56] 2015 (CJU)	Observational	40	Conductive	95	—	—	—	—	—
Sooriakumaran et al,[68] 2016	Observational	97	RITE	93	7	14	23	0	0
Kiss et al,[47] 2015	Observational	21	RITE	62	52	24	0	10	10
Sousa et al,[31] 2016	Observational	40	Conductive	98	8	23	23	3	3

Abbreviations: RITE, radiofrequency-induced thermo-chemotherapeutic effect; UTI, urinary tract infection.

Table 4
Clinical trials and observational studies on adjuvant intravesical MMC and EMDA

Author and Year Published	Trial	Sample Size	Treatment per Session	EMDA Device/Current	Induction Schedule	Maintenance Schedule for CR Group	Risk Group (% Patients)	Hx of Intravesical Therapy (% Patients)	Follow-up, Median (IQR)	1-y RFS	2-y RFS	5-y RFS
Di Stasi et al,[59] 2003	Phase III	36	40 mg MMC in 100 mL of distilled water for 60 min and EMDA	20 mA for 30 min	Once weekly ×6	Nonresponders: second induction course Responders: Once monthly ×10	High grade (100)	—	43 mo	100	66	38
		36	40 mg MMC in 100 mL of distilled water for 60 min	—	Once weekly ×6	Non-responders: second induction course Responders: Once monthly ×10	High grade (100)	—		100	62	34
		36	81 mg BCG in 50 mL saline for 120 min	—	Once weekly ×6	Nonresponders: second induction course Responders: Once monthly ×10	High grade (100)	—		100	39	21
Di Stasi et al,[60] 2006	Phase III	105	81 mg BCG for 120 min	—	Once weekly ×6	Once monthly × 10	High grade (100)	41	88 mo (63–110)	73	77	56
		107	(Week 1 and 2: 81 mg BCG for 120 min Week 3: 40 mg MMC in 100 mL of distilled water and EMDA) ×3	20 mA for 30 min	3 cycles (9 wk total)	Month 1, 2, 4, 5, 7, and 8: MMC + EMDA Months 3, 6, and 9: BCG	High grade (100)	42		100	49	40

(continued on next page)

Table 4
(continued)

Author and Year Published	Trial	Sample Size	Treatment per Session	EMDA Device/ Current	Induction Schedule	Maintenance Schedule for CR Group	Risk Group (% Patients)	Hx of Intravesical Therapy (% Patients)	Follow-up, Median (IQR)	1-y RFS	2-y RFS	5-y RFS
Di Stasi et al,[63] 2011	Phase III	124	TURBT	—	Once	Low-risk: none Intermediate risk: 40 mg MMC	High grade (82)	No previous intravesical treatment	92 mo (61–126)	62	42	37
		126	TURBT + immediate postoperative 40 mg MMC in 50 mL water for 60 min	—	Once	dissolved in 50 mL of sterile water for 60 min weekly ×6 High risk: 81 mg BCG dissolved in 50 mL	High grade (81)		82 mo (50–125)	65	47	43
		124	Neoadjuvant 40 mg MMC in 100 mL water for 30 min and EMDA + TURBT	20 mA for 30 min	Once	of saline for 120 min weekly ×6	High grade (82)		85 mo (57–126)	87	70	62
Riedl et al,[61] 1998	Observational	22	40 mg MMC in 100 mL saline	15 mA for 20 min	Once weekly ×4	—	High grade (95)	—	7.3 mo(mean)	—	—	—
Gan et al,[62] 2016	Observational	22	(Week 1 and 2: BCG Week 3: 40 mg MMC and EMDA) ×3	Physionizer ® 30: 20 mA for 30 min	3 cycles (9 wk total)	(Once weekly BCG) ×3 on month 3 and every 6 mo for 3 y	High grade (100)	—	24 mo	86	80	—

Dose in the maintenance group is similar to treatment unless stated otherwise.
Abbreviations: BCG, Bacillus Calmette-Guerin; CR, complete response; Hx, history; IQR, interquartile range; RFS, recurrence free survival; TURBT, transurethral resection of the bladder tumor.

and adjuvant settings (after TURBT). Intravesical EMDA MMC is administered using a controlled electric current of up to 30 mA using a battery-powered generator. A specialized 16 Fr catheter is inserted and urine drained. MMC is then instilled with an operating current of 15 to 20 mA pulsed electrical current for 20 to 30 minutes per session. To date, 2 small clinical trials have used EMDA in the neoadjuvant setting (**Table 3**) and 4 studies have used EMDA in the adjuvant setting (**Table 4**). EMDA was found to have a complete response rate of 40% in the neoadjuvant setting.[41,58] In the adjuvant setting, EMDA was found to have a 1-, 2-, and 5-year RFS rate of 86% to 100%, 49% to 80%, 38% to 40%, respectively.[59–62] One study evaluated TURBT, TURBT with immediate postoperative MMC and neoadjuvant MMC with EMDA followed by TURBT. Patients with intermediate-risk and high-risk disease in all 3 groups were then placed on maintenance MMC and BCG, respectively. The group that received neoadjuvant MMC with EMDA followed by TURBT had the highest 5-year RFS of 62% compared with 37% in the TURBT- only arm.[63]

Safety

The first bladder HT treatment was attempted in 1972 where Thiotepa was used in conjunction with HT up to 44°C for low stage bladder tumors.[64] Since then, multiple adverse events that include hematuria, urinary tract infection, sepsis, stricture, allergic reaction to chemotherapy agent, dysuria, frequency, urgency and incontinence have been reported (**Table 3**). There were insufficient data to pool for grade 3 or higher adverse events, urinary tract infection, sepsis, and allergic reaction. The rate of grade 3 or higher adverse event rate ranges from 10% to 12% across all sources of energy in patients receiving HT in clinical trials published.[31,65] Urinary tract infection and sepsis occurred in 0% to 23% of patients, and strictures in 0% to 10%.[65] Allergic reaction occurred in 0% to 15% of patients.[65] Pooling data for randomized controlled trials showed that the relative risk of hematuria in the HT arm is 1.28 (95% confidence interval, 0.89–1.83; $I^2 = 0$) when compared to the non-HT arm.

Future Perspectives and Other Novel Agents

For intermediate-risk NMIBC, HIVEC-I (EudraCT 2013–002628–18) and HIVEC-II (ISRCTN 23639415) are multi-institutional randomized controlled trials comparing HIVEC with standard MMC in patients with intermediate-risk NMIBC. Both trials have completed accrual (n = 598 subjects combined). HIVEC-HR (EudraCT 2016–

001186–85) is assessing HIVEC in high-risk NMIBC and HIVEC-R (EudraCT 2014–005001–20) is assessing HIVEC as neoadjuvant chemoablation. All of these trials are using the Combat BRS device. Lastly, the RITE-USA trial (NCT03335059) is assessing HT with the Synergo device for BCG-unresponsive NMIBC.

A novel temperature-sensitive liposome drug delivery system is worth highlighting here. The first drug, called ThermoDox is developed at Duke. It is loaded with doxorubicin and is administered systemically to releases free drug when it arrives in tissues heated to 41°C or greater. When combined with bladder HT, this technology allows for organ-specific targeting of systemic agents. In a swine model, Thermodox is able to achieve doxorubicin levels far exceeding free doxorubicin while minimizing toxicity in other organs.[66]

SUMMARY

Intravesical chemotherapy and HT therapy is safe and able to augment the efficacy of intravesical chemotherapy for the treatment of BCG refractory NMIBC, especially in a time of BCG shortage. Further prospective randomized controlled trials combining other forms of chemotherapy with HT therapy is warranted to determine if improved efficacy is obtained in those drugs. Other combinations of therapy such as combining HT and intravesical chemotherapy therapies such as programmed death-1/programmed death ligand 1 blockade is also warranted.

REFERENCES

1. Siegel RL, Miller KD, Jemal A. Cancer statistics, 2018. CA Cancer J Clin 2018;68(1):7–30.
2. Soloway MS. It is time to abandon the "superficial" in bladder cancer. Eur Urol 2007;52(6):1564–5.
3. National Comprehensive Cancer Network. Bladder Cancer (Version 1.2019). Available at: https://www.nccn.org/professionals/physician_gls/pdf/bladder.pdf. Accessed February 18, 2019.
4. Lamm DL, Blumenstein BA, Crissman JD, et al. Maintenance bacillus Calmette-Guerin immunotherapy for recurrent TA, T1 and carcinoma in situ transitional cell carcinoma of the bladder: a randomized Southwest Oncology Group Study. J Urol 2000; 163(4):1124–9.
5. Cambier S, Sylvester RJ, Collette L, et al. EORTC Nomograms and Risk Groups for predicting recurrence, progression, and disease-specific and overall survival in non-muscle-invasive stage Ta-T1 urothelial bladder cancer patients treated with 1-3 years of maintenance Bacillus Calmette-Guerin. Eur Urol 2016;69(1):60–9.

6. Kamat AM, Sylvester RJ, Bohle A, et al. Definitions, end points, and clinical trial designs for non-muscle-invasive bladder cancer: recommendations from the International Bladder Cancer Group. J Clin Oncol 2016;34(16):1935–44.

7. Falk MH, Issels RD. Hyperthermia in oncology. Int J Hyperthermia 2001;17(1):1–18.

8. Frey B, Weiss EM, Rubner Y, et al. Old and new facts about hyperthermia-induced modulations of the immune system. Int J Hyperthermia 2012;28(6):528–42.

9. Hildebrandt B, Wust P, Ahlers O, et al. The cellular and molecular basis of hyperthermia. Crit Rev Oncol Hematol 2002;43(1):33–56.

10. Wust P, Hildebrandt B, Sreenivasa G, et al. Hyperthermia in combined treatment of cancer. Lancet Oncol 2002;3(8):487–97.

11. Issels RD. Hyperthermia adds to chemotherapy. Eur J Cancer 2008;44(17):2546–54.

12. Maeda H, Tsukigawa K, Fang J. A retrospective 30 years after discovery of the enhanced permeability and retention effect of solid tumors: next-generation chemotherapeutics and photodynamic therapy–problems, solutions, and prospects. Microcirculation 2016;23(3):173–82.

13. Vaupel P, Kallinowski F, Okunieff P. Blood flow, oxygen and nutrient supply, and metabolic microenvironment of human tumors: a review. Cancer Res 1989;49(23):6449–65.

14. Song CW. Effect of local hyperthermia on blood flow and microenvironment: a review. Cancer Res 1984;44(10 Supplement):4721s–30s.

15. Robinson JE, Wizenberg MJ, McCready WA. Radiation and hyperthermal response of normal tissue in situ. Radiology 1974;113(1):195–8.

16. Takemoto M, Kuroda M, Urano M, et al. The effect of various chemotherapeutic agents given with mild hyperthermia on different types of tumours. Int J Hyperthermia 2003;19(2):193–203.

17. Vertrees RA, Das GC, Popov VL, et al. Synergistic interaction of hyperthermia and Gemcitabine in lung cancer. Cancer Biol Ther 2005;4(10):1144–53.

18. Zhang HG, Mehta K, Cohen P, et al. Hyperthermia on immune regulation: a temperature's story. Cancer Lett 2008;271(2):191–204.

19. Evans SS, Repasky EA, Fisher DT. Fever and the thermal regulation of immunity: the immune system feels the heat. Nat Rev Immunol 2015;15(6):335–49.

20. Milani V, Noessner E, Ghose S, et al. Heat shock protein 70: role in antigen presentation and immune stimulation. Int J Hyperthermia 2002;18(6):563–75.

21. Longo TA, Gopalakrishna A, Tsivian M, et al. A systematic review of regional hyperthermia therapy in bladder cancer. Int J Hyperthermia 2016;32(4):381–9.

22. van der Zee J, Gonzalez Gonzalez D, van Rhoon GC, et al. Comparison of radiotherapy alone with radiotherapy plus hyperthermia in locally advanced pelvic tumours: a prospective, randomised, multicentre trial. Dutch Deep Hyperthermia Group. Lancet 2000;355(9210):1119–25.

23. Wittlinger M, Rodel CM, Weiss C, et al. Quadrimodal treatment of high-risk T1 and T2 bladder cancer: transurethral tumor resection followed by concurrent radiochemotherapy and regional deep hyperthermia. Radiother Oncol 2009;93(2):358–63.

24. Inman BA, Stauffer PR, Craciunescu OA, et al. A pilot clinical trial of intravesical mitomycin-C and external deep pelvic hyperthermia for non-muscle-invasive bladder cancer. Int J Hyperthermia 2014;30(3):171–5.

25. Petrovich Z, Emami B, Kapp D, et al. Regional hyperthermia in patients with recurrent genitourinary cancer. Am J Clin Oncol 1991;14(6):472–7.

26. Sapozink MD, Gibbs FA Jr, Egger MJ, et al. Regional hyperthermia for clinically advanced deep-seated pelvic malignancy. Am J Clin Oncol 1986;9(2):162–9.

27. Crezee J, Van Haaren PM, Westendorp H, et al. Improving locoregional hyperthermia delivery using the 3-D controlled AMC-8 phased array hyperthermia system: a preclinical study. Int J Hyperthermia 2009;25(7):581–92.

28. Geijsen ED, de Reijke TM, Koning CC, et al. Combining mitomycin C and regional 70 MHz hyperthermia in patients with nonmuscle invasive bladder cancer: a pilot study. J Urol 2015;194(5):1202–8.

29. Rietbroek RC, Bakker PJ, Schilthuis MS, et al. Feasibility, toxicity, and preliminary results of weekly locoregional hyperthermia and cisplatin in patients with previously irradiated recurrent cervical carcinoma or locally advanced bladder cancer. Int J Radiat Oncol Biol Phys 1996;34(4):887–93.

30. de Castro Abreu AL, Ukimura O, Shoji S, et al. Robotic transmural ablation of bladder tumors using high-intensity focused ultrasound: experimental study. Int J Urol 2016;23(6):501–8.

31. Sousa A, Pineiro I, Rodriguez S, et al. Recirculant hyperthermic IntraVEsical chemotherapy (HIVEC) in intermediate-high-risk non-muscle-invasive bladder cancer. Int J Hyperthermia 2016;32(4):374–80.

32. Soria F, Milla P, Fiorito C, et al. Efficacy and safety of a new device for intravesical thermochemotherapy in non-grade 3 BCG recurrent NMIBC: a phase I-II study. World J Urol 2016;34(2):189–95.

33. Colombo R, Salonia A, Leib Z, et al. Long-term outcomes of a randomized controlled trial comparing thermochemotherapy with mitomycin-C alone as adjuvant treatment for non-muscle-invasive bladder cancer (NMIBC). BJU Int 2011;107(6):912–8.

34. Gofrit ON, Shapiro A, Pode D, et al. Combined local bladder hyperthermia and intravesical chemotherapy for the treatment of high-grade superficial bladder cancer. Urology 2004;63(3):466–71.

35. Rigatti P, Lev A, Colombo R. Combined intravesical chemotherapy with mitomycin C and local bladder microwave-induced hyperthermia as a preoperative therapy for superficial bladder tumors. A preliminary clinical study. Eur Urol 1991;20(3):204–10.

36. Jung JH, Gudeloglu A, Kiziloz H, et al. Intravesical electromotive drug administration for non-muscle invasive bladder cancer. Cochrane Database Syst Rev 2017;(9):CD011864.

37. Oliveira TR, Stauffer PR, Lee CT, et al. Magnetic fluid hyperthermia for bladder cancer: a preclinical dosimetry study. Int J Hyperthermia 2013;29(8):835–44.

38. Sousa A, Inman BA, Pineiro I, et al. A clinical trial of neoadjuvant hyperthermic intravesical chemotherapy (HIVEC) for treating intermediate and high-risk non-muscle invasive bladder cancer. Int J Hyperthermia 2014;30(3):166–70.

39. Colombo R, Lev A, Da Pozzo LF, et al. A new approach using local combined microwave hyperthermia and chemotherapy in superficial transitional bladder carcinoma treatment. J Urol 1995;153(3 Pt 2):959–63.

40. Colombo R, Da Pozzo LF, Lev A, et al. Neoadjuvant combined microwave induced local hyperthermia and topical chemotherapy versus chemotherapy alone for superficial bladder cancer. J Urol 1996; 155(4):1227–32.

41. Colombo R, Colombo R, Brausi M, et al. Thermo–chemotherapy and electromotive drug administration of mitomycin C in superficial bladder cancer eradication. Eur Urol 2001;39(1):95–100.

42. van der Heijden AG, Kiemeney LA, Gofrit ON, et al. Preliminary European results of local microwave hyperthermia and chemotherapy treatment in intermediate or high risk superficial transitional cell carcinoma of the bladder. Eur Urol 2004;46(1):65–71 [discussion: 71–2].

43. Colombo R, Da Pozzo LF, Salonia A, et al. Multicentric study comparing intravesical chemotherapy alone and with local microwave hyperthermia for prophylaxis of recurrence of superficial transitional cell carcinoma. J Clin Oncol 2003;21(23):4270–6.

44. Arends TJ, Nativ O, Maffezzini M, et al. Results of a randomised controlled trial comparing intravesical chemohyperthermia with mitomycin C versus Bacillus Calmette-Guerin for adjuvant treatment of patients with intermediate- and high-risk non-muscle-invasive bladder cancer. Eur Urol 2016;69(6):1046–52.

45. Tan WS, Panchal A, Buckley L, et al. Radiofrequency-induced thermo-chemotherapy effect versus a second course of Bacillus Calmette-Guerin or institutional standard in patients with recurrence of non-muscle-invasive bladder cancer following induction or maintenance Bacillus Calmette-Guerin therapy (HYMN): a phase III, open-label, randomised controlled trial. Eur Urol 2019;75(1):63–71.

46. Arends TJ, van der Heijden AG, Witjes JA. Combined chemohyperthermia: 10-year single center experience in 160 patients with nonmuscle invasive bladder cancer. J Urol 2014;192(3):708–13.

47. Kiss B, Schneider S, Thalmann GN, et al. Is thermo-chemotherapy with the Synergo system a viable treatment option in patients with recurrent non-muscle-invasive bladder cancer? Int J Urol 2015; 22(2):158–62.

48. Moskovitz B, Meyer G, Kravtzov A, et al. Thermo-chemotherapy for intermediate or high-risk recurrent superficial bladder cancer patients. Ann Oncol 2005;16(4):585–9.

49. Alfred Witjes J, Hendricksen K, Gofrit O, et al. Intravesical hyperthermia and mitomycin-C for carcinoma in situ of the urinary bladder: experience of the European Synergo working party. World J Urol 2009;27(3):319–24.

50. Moskovitz B, Halachmi S, Moskovitz M, et al. 10-year single-center experience of combined intravesical chemohyperthermia for nonmuscle invasive bladder cancer. Future Oncol 2012;8(8):1041–9.

51. Volpe A, Racioppi M, Bongiovanni L, et al. Thermo-chemotherapy for non-muscle-invasive bladder cancer: is there a chance to avoid early cystectomy? Urol Int 2012;89(3):311–8.

52. Nativ O, Witjes JA, Hendricksen K, et al. Combined thermo-chemotherapy for recurrent bladder cancer after Bacillus Calmette-Guerin. J Urol 2009;182(4):1313–7.

53. Halachmi S, Moskovitz B, Maffezzini M, et al. Intravesical mitomycin C combined with hyperthermia for patients with T1G3 transitional cell carcinoma of the bladder. Urol Oncol 2011;29(3):259–64.

54. Maffezzini M, Campodonico F, Canepa G, et al. Intravesical mitomycin C combined with local microwave hyperthermia in non-muscle-invasive bladder cancer with increased European Organization for Research and Treatment of Cancer (EORTC) score risk of recurrence and progression. Cancer Chemother Pharmacol 2014;73(5):925–30.

55. Ekin RG, Akarken I, Cakmak O, et al. Results of intravesical chemo-hyperthermia in high-risk non-muscle invasive bladder cancer. Asian Pac J Cancer Prev 2015;16(8):3241–5.

56. Ekin RG, Akarken I, Zorlu F, et al. Intravesical Bacillus Calmette-Guerin versus chemohyperthermia for high-risk non-muscle-invasive bladder cancer. Can Urol Assoc J 2015;9(5–6):E278–83.

57. Sooriakumaran P, Chiocchia V, Dutton S, et al. Predictive factors for time to progression after hyperthermic mitomycin C treatment for high-risk non-muscle invasive urothelial carcinoma of the bladder: an observational cohort study of 97 patients. Urol Int 2016;96(1):83–90.

58. Brausi M, Campo B, Pizzocaro G, et al. Intravesical electromotive administration of drugs for treatment of superficial bladder cancer: a comparative Phase II study. Urology 1998;51(3):506–9.

59. Di Stasi SM, Giannantoni A, Stephen RL, et al. Intravesical electromotive mitomycin C versus passive transport mitomycin C for high risk superficial bladder cancer: a prospective randomized study. J Urol 2003;170(3):777–82.

60. Di Stasi SM, Giannantoni A, Giurioli A, et al. Sequential BCG and electromotive mitomycin versus BCG alone for high-risk superficial bladder cancer: a randomised controlled trial. Lancet Oncol 2006; 7(1):43–51.

61. Riedl CR, Knoll M, Plas E, et al. Intravesical electromotive drug administration technique: preliminary results and side effects. J Urol 1998;159(6):1851–6.

62. Gan C, Amery S, Chatterton K, et al. Sequential Bacillus Calmette-Guerin/electromotive drug administration of mitomycin C as the standard intravesical regimen in high risk nonmuscle invasive bladder cancer: 2-year outcomes. J Urol 2016; 195(6):1697–703.

63. Di Stasi SM, Valenti M, Verri C, et al. Electromotive instillation of mitomycin immediately before transurethral resection for patients with primary urothelial non-muscle invasive bladder cancer: a randomised controlled trial. Lancet Oncol 2011;12(9):871–9.

64. Lunglmayr G, Czech K, Zekert F, et al. Bladder hyperthermia in the treatment of vesical papillomatosis. Int Urol Nephrol 1973;5(1):75–84.

65. Tan WS, Kelly JD. Intravesical device-assisted therapies for non-muscle-invasive bladder cancer. Nat Rev Urol 2018;15(11):667–85.

66. Brousell SC, Longo TA, Fantony JJ, et al. MP65-08 heat-targeted drug delivery using the combat brs device for treating bladder cancer. J Urol 2017; 197(4, Supplement):e855.

67. Halachmi S, Moskovitz B, Maffezzini M, et al. Intravesical mitomycin C combined with hyperthermia for patients with T1G3 transitional cell carcinoma of the bladder. Urol Oncol 2011 May-Jun;29(3): 259–64. https://doi.org/10.1016/j.urolonc.2009.02. 012.

68. Sooriakumaran P, Chiocchia V, Dutton S, et al. Predictive Factors for Time to Progression after Hyperthermic Mitomycin C Treatment for High-Risk Non-Muscle Invasive Urothelial Carcinoma of the Bladder: An Observational Cohort Study of 97 Patients. Urol Int 2016;96(1):83–90. https://doi.org/10. 1159/000435788.

Apaziquone for Nonmuscle Invasive Bladder Cancer
Where Are We Now?

Tom J.H. Arends, PhD[a], Johannes Alfred Witjes, PhD[b],*

KEYWORDS

• Apaziquone • Bladder cancer • Nonmuscle invasive • Therapy • Experimental

KEY POINTS

• Apaziquone is an interesting drug for intravesical use in patients with nonmuscle invasive bladder cancer; however, more research is needed to prove its actual benefit.
• Although the apaziquone trials demonstrate the potential of this new drug, the singular phase 3 trials did not reach their primary endpoint.
• To date, no new trials are recruiting, the development of apaziquone seems to have stopped.

INTRODUCTION

Bladder cancer (BC) is the second most common genitourinary malignancy worldwide and has a great impact on health care infrastructure and costs.[1,2] Worldwide, approximately 2.7 million patients have been diagnosed, treated, and followed for BC at any given time point.[1,3] Seventy-five percent of BC patients present with nonmuscle invasive bladder cancer (NMIBC). BC presents with macroscopic hematuria in most cases. Risk factors are predominantly smoking and some industrial exposures like aromatic aromines and dyes. There is a 3 to 4 to 1 male predominance.[4]

NMIBC is characterized by a high recurrence rate, which emphasizes the need for adjuvant intravesical therapies after transurethral resection (TURBT). To date, intravesical chemotherapy for low- and intermediate-risk tumors and intravesical *Bacillus Calmette-Guerin* (BCG) therapy for intermediate- and high-risk tumors are the gold standards. Despite adjuvant treatment, however, up to 61% of all patients will recur within 1 year.[5,6] Particularly in patients with high risk NMIBC, the risk of progression also increases, and because of the lack of alternative conservative treatments, this may result in early cystectomy.

In low-risk patients, a single adjuvant chemotherapeutic instillation is sufficient. This advice is predominantly based on large meta-analysis, comparing transurethral resection of a bladder tumor (TURBT) alone to TURBT plus 1 immediate instillation of chemotherapy.[7] Seven randomized trials with 1476 patients and a median follow-up of 3.4 years were analyzed. Two hundred sixty-seven (36.7%) of 728 patients recurred after TURBT and 1 instillation with chemotherapy compared to 362 (48.4%) of the 748 patients treated with TURBT alone (odds ratio [OR] 0.61, *P*<.0001). Patients with single tumors (OR 0.61) and multiple tumors (OR 0.44) benefited. However, because 65.2% of patients with multiple tumors had a recurrence after this 1 instillation, compared to 35.8% of patients with single tumors, the authors concluded that 1 instillation alone was insufficient for multiple tumors. It is, therefore, the treatment of choice in patients with single, low-risk papillary

Disclosures: Dr J.A. Witjes was a previous advisor of Spectrum Pharmaceuticals (until 2017) and primary investigator in apaziquone studies.

[a] Department of Urology, Canisius Wilhelmina Hospital, Weg door Jonkerbos 100, 6532 SZ Nijmegen, The Netherlands; [b] Department of Urology, Radboud University Nijmegen Medical Centre, Geert Groote plein zuid 10, 6525 GA Nijmegen, The Netherlands
* Corresponding author.
E-mail address: fred.witjes@radboudumc.nl

Urol Clin N Am 47 (2020) 73–82
https://doi.org/10.1016/j.ucl.2019.09.009

tumors. Furthermore, no difference between the chemotherapeutic drugs used could be found. The instillation should probably be given within 6 hours after operation, but in any case within 24 hours, unless there has been a bladder perforation or extensive/deep resection.[7]

In high-risk patients, a second TURBT is mandatory, as residual or recurrent disease within 3 months after TURBT for NMIBC can be up to 45%.[8–12] Therefore, a second TURBT within 2 to 4 weeks is strongly recommended by the current guidelines.[4]

For these high-risk patients, additional therapy consists of intravesical Bacillus Calmette-Guérin (BCG). BCG is superior to any other adjuvant intravesical drug in the prevention of recurrence of NMIBC, and it is considered to prevent and/or delay progression of NMIBC.

A large meta-analysis showed that BCG had a lower risk of tumor progression in comparison to intravesical chemotherapy.[13] Twenty-four trials with 4863 patients and a median follow-up of 2.5 years were reported. Two hundred sixty (9.8%) of 2658 patients on BCG had progression as compared to 304 (13.8%) of 2205 patients without BCG (OR = 0.73, $P=.001$). This effect was similar in patients with papillary tumors and in those with carcinoma in situ (CIS), but only patients receiving maintenance BCG benefited. Limitations of this study are the overall low percentage of progression (6.4% of 2880 patients with papillary tumors and 13.9% of 403 patients with CIS) as a result of the short follow-up and relatively favorable patient profile. Last, but not least, no significant difference in disease-specific survival was found. A disadvantage of BCG is that it has more severe local and systemic adverse effects compared with chemotherapy. When patients fail on BCG, radical cystectomy is the safest option.[4,14] Adjuvant intravesical treatment in these patients remains experimental.

For the largest group of patients, the intermediate-risk group of NMIBC, intravesical chemotherapeutic instillations can reduce the risk of recurrence. However, in the long term, it only causes a modest reduction of the risk of recurrence, without reduction in the risk of progression. In a combined analysis of individual patient data from previously performed EORTC (European Organisation for Research and Treatment of Cancer) and Medical Research Council (MRC) randomized trials, including a total of 2535 patients, the effect of adjuvant intravesical chemotherapy or adjuvant oral agents on several endpoints in TaT1 NMIBC was calculated.[15] Only the disease-free survival was significantly prolonged after adjuvant treatment compared with no adjuvant treatment ($P<.01$). Still, the differences were modest. For example, the disease-free estimate at 8 years was 44.9% in the treatment group, versus 36.7% in the no treatment group. No significant or relevant advantage was shown for progression to invasive or metastatic disease, or duration of (progression-free) survival.[15] In case of recurrent intermediate-risk NMIBC, additional chemotherapeutic instillations or instillations with BCG are advocated.[16,17]

In conclusion, initial therapy of NMIBC is TURBT, followed by intravesical therapy with chemotherapeutic drugs or BCG. The choice of drugs, frequency, and schedule used for these additional intravesical instillations are defined by guidelines. However, therapy is not without toxicity, and a substantial percentage of treated patients still experience tumor recurrences or progression to muscle-invasive bladder cancer (MIBC), so several unmet needs remain.

This article reports on the developments of new intravesical therapies and strategies, with a main focus on the mitomycin (MMC)-derivative apaziquone. In 2008, the first review considering apaziquone was published in Expert Opinion on Investigational Drugs by the same research group.[16] New data and insights are added considering the current status of apaziquone in 2019.

The Impact on Health Care

Botteman and colleagues[18–39] looked at health economics related to BC. They calculated that BC is the fifth most expensive cancer, but considering the (life) long surveillance, the per patient costs for BC from diagnosis until death appeared to be highest of all cancers.

In conclusion, NMIBC is a highly recurrent disease with a tremendous impact on patients, doctors, and health care costs.

NEW INTRAVESICAL TREATMENTS FOR NONMUSCLE-INVASIVE BLADDER CANCER

The high amount of recurrence in NMIBC patients stresses the need for new intravesical therapies and strategies. Several new therapies are under study; however, none has been implanted as standard therapy yet. In this article, the authors focus on the relatively new agent apaziquone.

Bacillus Calmette-Guerin Failures

In the European Association of Urology (EAU) guidelines, BCG treatment failure is defined as

   Muscular invasion, detected during follow-up
   The presence of high-grade NMIBC at both 3 and 6 months after initial treatment

Any deterioration of the disease under BCG treatment, such as a higher number of recurrences, higher T stage or higher grade, or the appearance of CIS, despite an initial response[4]

In daily practice, a subdivision of BCG failure patients into 4 groups can be used:

1. Patients intolerant because of adverse effects
2. BCG resistance that includes recurrence/persistence of lesser disease and which resolves with further BCG
3. BCG-relapsing patients, which means recurrence after initial resolution
4. BCG-refractory disease (those patients primarily not improving or even worsening under BCG treatment)

BCG intolerance is inevitable, with various clinical studies reporting recurrence rates of 20% to 53% within 5 years and progression rates of up to 28%.[40] In BCG-intolerant patients, certainly in those who never completed the induction course, intravesical therapy with another drug at the time of recurrence is worth trying.[14]

BCG induces a 70% initial complete response rate, which remains in 50% after long follow-up. Around 40% to 60% of the initial nonresponders will respond to a second course of BCG.[41–44] Real failures are those patients having a recurrence during BCG treatment or those who are not achieving a complete response. Unfortunately, one cannot to predict BCG failure accurately on an individual basis. However, with clinical and histologic parameters, risk groups can and should be identified, because the window of opportunity is limited; in case of tumor progression to MIBC, the survival rate drops dramatically, and the outcome is far worse than in primary MIBC patients. In a recent systematic review of 19 trials (total of 3088 patients), progression to MIBC was seen in 21%, of which 14% died of BC after a follow-up of 48 to 123 months. Hence, the long-term cancer-specific survival after progression was as low as 37%.[45]

Therefore, the EAU treatment guidelines recommend the consideration of cystectomy after initial BCG failure in patients with high-grade recurrences.[4] The advantage is obvious, as early cystectomy in BCG failure patients is associated with a recurrence-free 5-year survival rate of 80% to 90%.[46] On the other hand, some of these patients will be overtreated, and become disadvantaged by the comorbidity, mortality, and impaired quality of life associated with this procedure.[47]

Apaziquone

Apaziquone, a quinone-based bioreductive drug, was originally developed by the Netherlands Cancer Institute. Its preclinical and systemic early clinical studies were conducted within the EORTC framework.

Despite reports of 3 partial responses in phase 1 studies, no responses were seen in phase 2 clinical trials with intravenous apaziquone. It was hypothesized that the rapid pharmacokinetic elimination and relatively poor penetration of the drug could have compromised drug delivery to tumors following systemic administration.[48]

If this is the case, these unfavorable pharmacokinetic properties of intravenous administration could be turned to an advantage for apaziquone in the treatment of cancers in third compartments like the urinary bladder. Subsequent studies confirmed that NMIBC cases have elevated levels of the activating enzyme DT-diaphorase (DTD). Apaziquone (EOquin) is a prodrug that is activated by DTD and other reductases to generate cytotoxicity that leads to apoptosis. Apaziquone has potent antitumor activity, proven in both in vitro and in vivo tumor models.[49,50]

Apaziquone is chemically composed as 5-(aziridin-1-yl)-3-(hydroxymethyl)-2-[(1E)-3-hydroxyprop-1-enyl]-1-methyl-1H-indole-4,7-dione. Its molecular formula is $C_{15}H_{16}N_2O$. The molecular weight of apaziquone is 288.30 kDa. The drug product EOquin (apaziquone for intravesical instillation) is supplied as a sterile, nonpyrogenic lyophilized product in clear glass vials. It contains 4 mg apaziquone, as well as mannitol and sodium bicarbonate. The recommended storage temperature is 2° to 8°C. Prior to intravesical instillation, the EOquin vial is reconstituted with 20 mL of "Diluent for EOquin" (a propylene glycol solution for intravesical instillation), to yield 0.2 mg/mL of apaziquone. This solution is further diluted with 20 mL of sterile water for injection, resulting in 40 mL of the instillation solution containing 0.1 mg/mL of apaziquone.[16]

Preclinical activity

The antitumor activity of apaziquone has been evaluated in murine tumor models and in human tumor lines, both in vitro and in vivo.

Cytotoxicity against various tumor cell lines was evaluated by different investigators.[51] Apaziquone is highly cytotoxic against a broad spectrum of cell lines, and it inhibits the growth of most cell lines tested at nanomolar concentrations. Of note, in vitro apaziquone potency was a multiple of that of MMC in most solid tumors, achieving a mean 50% growth inhibitory concentration of 17 nm against 710 nm for MMC.[52]

In the cytotoxicity studies, the mean graphs of apaziquone show a characteristic pattern with clusters of sensitive cell lines derived from colon, melanoma, and central nervous system (CNS) tumors. Unlike MMC, apaziquone showed preferential cytotoxicity against solid tumors and was much less active or inactive against most leukemia. This was also evident from the Corbett 2-tumor assay. No activity in leukemias was seen in the human tumor line screen either, where apaziquone was assayed over a broad concentration range against a panel of 56 cell lines and displayed substantial potency in most of the available sensitive lines of colon, melanoma, renal, and CNS tumors. Noteworthy is the lack of significant differences in apaziquone sensitivity between MCF-7 (breast adenocarcinoma) and its derivative expressing the multidrug resistance phenotype MCF-7/ADR.[51]

Continuous exposure of cells from subcutaneously growing human tumors in a colony-forming assay in nude mice showed high sensitivity to apaziquone in breast, colon, nonsmall cell lung and kidney cancer lines.

In an in vitro test against 4 small-cell lung cancer cell lines, both with 1-hour incubation and with continuous exposure, a small increase in potency with increased exposure time suggested that apaziquone activity is not cell cycle specific.

Aerobic cytotoxicity analysis of apaziquone and MMC against EMT6 mouse breast cancer line after either 1 hour or continuous exposure was done by MTT dye reduction. Apaziquone was tenfold to 20-fold more potent than MMC against this cell line. Apaziquone cytotoxicity under hypoxic versus oxic conditions was compared in a clonogenic assay in EMT6 mouse mammary tumor cells using a 3-hour exposure experiment. Concentrations required to reduce cell survival to 10% of control were 3 and 10 ng/mL (ratio 3.3) for hypoxic and oxic cells, respectively.[16]

In human tumor xenografts, apaziquone induced tumor regression in gastric cancer GXF 97 and ovarian cancer MRI-H-207. A single intravenous injection of 2 mg/kg MMC, however, caused tumor regression in GXF 97 (T/C 5.3%), and in MRI-H-207, 2 weekly intravenous injections of 5 mg/kg induced complete remissions A third injection of apaziquone in MRI-H-207-bearing nude mice induced almost complete remissions. Growth delay in breast cancer MAXF 449 and marginal activity in the nonsmall cell lung cancer LXFL 529 were seen. No antitumor activity was found in the renal cancer RXF 243.[16]

In conclusion, apaziquone is a potent cytotoxic agent preferentially active in solid tumor lines.

Pharmacokinetics and metabolism

Pharmacokinetics of intravenous injection in rodents and dogs using a high-performance liquid chromatography (HPLC) method show that clearance is rapid and the half-life short (1.9 minutes in the mouse, 3 minutes in the rat at nontoxic doses and 4–14 minutes in the dog). The half-life is linear in the mouse and rat, but not the dog, in which it shows a beta phase. Area under the curve increased with the dose, and maximal plasma concentrations after intravenous administration of 0.41 to 1.64 mg/kg were in the 0.6 to 1 µg/mL range in the dog. Two major metabolites appear in the plasma, along with several minor peaks. Apaziquone was not found in the urine, which contained numerous metabolites. In any case, the drug is extensively and rapidly metabolized.[53]

In the human studies of intravenous administration, the pharmacokinetics of apaziquone were determined in 32 and 28 patients, treated in phase 1 studies of apaziquone given every 3 weeks or weekly.[54,55] The recommended doses reached were 22 mg/m^2 every 3 weeks and 12 mg/m^2 weekly. The plasma curve fit a 2-compartment model. Pharmacokinetic parameters varied widely between patients; the half-life, however, was almost uniformly short (mean 10 minutes).[16]

Intravesical instillation in animal studies
Apaziquone at a concentration 4 and 16 times higher than that used in the human phase 2 trial (0.1 mg/mL) was instilled into the urinary bladder of 4 Beagle dogs in a range-finding pilot toxicology study in 2 dogs at each of the 2 levels. The maximum plasma concentration reached with the higher dose concentration of 1.6 mg/mL was 21 ng/mL as detected by liquid chromatography/mass spectrometry (LC-MS). This level is considerably lower than the maximal concentrations that had been reported after administration of nontoxic intravenous doses to Beagles.[54]

A second study in dogs, with 6 weekly instillations at drug concentrations of 0.0125, 0.05, and 0.2 mg/mL, used the same analytical methods, with a lower limit of quantitation of 5 ng/mL in the dog plasma.[54] Out of 237 samples drawn after the start of instillation, 7 showed apaziquone levels above the lower limit of quantitation (5.4–75.5 ng/mL) and none above 20 ng/mL (lower limit of quantitation) for metabolite EO5a. It was concluded that penetration into the blood flow from the intact bladder is absent or minimal.

Phase 1/2 safety studies

During the phase 1/2 study of intravesical instillation 2 weeks after TURBT, blood and urine were collected in all instillation treatments in the 6 patients of the first intrapatient dose escalation cohort and in the 6 patients of the fixed-dose treatment cohort during and after the first and last instillations only.[56]

Blood was collected before treatment, and 30 and 55 minutes after the start of instillation. Bladder contents were drained at the end of the instillation and the samples buffered and frozen. Analysis of the samples was by HPLC with a lower limit of quantitation of 20 ng/mL. No apaziquone or its metabolite EO5 was detected in the plasma samples. Apaziquone was found in the bladder contents at the end of the 1-hour instillation, and its concentration increased linearly with the dose. The pH of bladder contents was relatively consistent (6.80 ± 0.84–7.66 ± 0.59), and percentage drug recovery after 1 hour was similar for all doses administered, accounting for 57.1 plus or minus 27.6 to 72.0 plus or minus 3.67% of the dose administered. The volume of bladder contents at the end of each instillation varied considerably, with values ranging from 112.5 plus or minus 40.6 to 240.0 plus or minus 112.2 mL. This may be dose-dependent, although considerable variation in the volume of instillation occurs at all doses administered.[56]

During the pilot study of immediate post-TURBT instillation, blood samples were collected from 6 of the 23 patients, before instillation and at 5, 15, 30, 45, and 60 minutes from its start. The samples were analyzed by a sensitive LC-MS method with a lower limit of quantitation of 5 ng/mL.[57]

The possibility of intravesical instillation reaching toxic levels of apaziquone or metabolites in the blood seems low, considering that the total dose recommended for instillation, 4 mg, is the equivalent of 20% of the tolerated weekly intravenous dose in an average patient with 1.7 m^2 BSA.[55]

In conclusion, apaziquone was ineffective by systemic administration probably because of its rapid elimination; it is not absorbed from the bladder even when instilled within 6 hours from TURBT, and its toxic potential, even if entirely absorbed, remains low.

Dose-finding/marker lesion studies

In preclinical research the concentration of apaziquone needed to achieve 50% cell kill at 37°C was 6 to 78 times lower than that of MMC depending on the cancer cell line used.[58]

In a dose-finding study, Puri and colleagues[56] determined the dose of apaziquone that could safely be administered in the bladder in patients with NMIBC. Six patients with multifocal, Ta/T1, and G1/G2 urothelial cell carcinoma received escalating doses of apaziquone (0.5 mg/40 mL up to 16 mg/40 mL) weekly for 6 weeks after resection of all but 1 lesion (the marker lesion). An additional 6 patients received weekly apaziquone in the highest nontoxic dose established. Pharmacokinetic parameters were determined in urine and blood, and the pharmacodynamic markers NQO1 (reduced nicotinamide adenine dinucleotide phosphate:quinone oxidoreductase-1) and glucose transporter 1 were also characterized. Local toxicity (grades 2 and 3 dysuria and hematuria) was observed at doses of 8 and 16 mg/40 mL, but 4 mg/40 mL were well tolerated with no systemic or local adverse effects. Urinary apaziquone increased linearly with the dose, but no apaziquone was detected in plasma. In 8 of 12 patients, complete macroscopic and histologic disappearance of the marker lesion occurred. A correlation between response and pharmacokinetic measurements could not be found.[56]

Van der Heijden and colleagues[58] performed a subsequent phase 2 marker lesion study on 46 patients with Ta-T1 G1-G2 NMIBC undergoing TURBT, with the exception of 1 marker lesion of 0.5 to 1 cm. Six weekly intravesical EOquin instillations of 4 mg/40 mL were administered. The adverse effects of EOquin in this study were comparable to other chemotherapeutic agents used against NMIBC, and the histologically proven complete response 2 to 4 weeks after the last instillation was 67% (30/45 patients). The remaining patient, who did not receive all 6 instillations, also had a compete response of the marker lesion.[58]

In conclusion, these 2 initial studies clearly show that apaziquone is safe and has a marked effect on marker lesions.

Phase 2/3 efficacy trials (2009–2018)

In 2009, an update the 2 year follow-up was published of this phase 2 marker lesion study by Hendricksen and colleagues.[59] The objective was to study the time to recurrence and duration of response of the same cohort from Van der Heijden and colleagues[58] in 2006. Routine follow-up was performed at 6, 9, 12, 18, and 24 months from the first apaziquone intstillation. The authors found that in an intention-to-treat analysis (2 complete response patients dropped out during follow-up) 49.5% of the complete responders remained recurrence free at 24 months of follow-up. The median duration of response was 18 months. Of the 15 nonresponders, only 2 had additional prophylactic instillations after TURBT. Of the nonresponders, 26.7% were recurrence free without additional intravesical therapies except for the additional TURBT to remove the remaining marker lesion. One nonresponding patient progressed to muscle-invasive disease. Adverse effects did not exceed grade 3, and no clinical meaningful changes were found by blood chemistry and/or urinalysis.[59]

The same research group presented a new phase 2 study in 2012. In this multicentre prospective phase 2 trial that was conducted in 3 Dutch hospitals, the efficacy and safety of multiple adjuvant apaziquone instillations were studied in patients with high-risk NMIBC.[60] Fifty-three patients with high-risk NMIBC were enrolled and underwent TURBT of all lesions and 6 weekly adjuvant intravesical apaziquone instillations of 4 mg in 40 mL. Follow-up with cystoscopy, cytology, and adverse events was executed every 3 months, for 18 months in total. In the intention-to-treat analysis, 34.7% and 44.9% of the patients recurred at 12 and 18 months, respectively. One patient had progression to muscle-invasive disease at the 9-month follow-up. Adverse effects were mild, with mostly grade 1 to 2 reported by the investigators. No systemic toxicity was observed.[60]

Noteworthy, the guideline definitions of intermediate- and high-risk BC changed during the conduct of this study. Although all patients were high risk according to the definitions when included in this trial, according to the most recent guideline criteria, 80% of the population would now be considered intermediate risk.

In 2018, 2 parallel phase 3, double-blind, placebo-controlled multinational trials were published in 1 extensive paper. These studies were performed following a Special Protocol Agreement with the US Food and Drug Administration (FDA). These 2 nearly identical trials (SPI-611 and SPI-612) were conducted between April 2007 and January 2012. Their objective was to evaluate the 2-year recurrence rate on time to recurrence in a Ta,G1-G2 randomized cohort receiving complete TURBT plus apaziquone versus TURBT plus placebo. A single intravesical instillation of apaziquone (4 mg/40 mL) or placebo was administered within 6 hours after TURBT.[61]

Researchers enrolled 1614 patients, of whom 1146 patients met the histologic inclusion criteria after TURBT. In both studies, the primary endpoints were not met, although the studies showed 6.7% and 6.6% reduction recurrence in the apaziquone group (not significant compared with the placebo group). When combined, the pooled analysis did show a significant reduction in the 2-year recurrence rate of 6.7% (OR 0.76;

P=.0218). In both studies, the time to recurrence showed improvement in the apaziquone group. In the SPI-611 study, this improvement was significant; in the SPI-612 study it was not. Pooled data for time to recurrence, again, did show significant improvement of time-to-recurrence (hazard ratio [HR] 0.79; P=.0096). The authors performed a post hoc analysis that showed that apaziquone instilled within 30 minutes after TURBT provided no benefit in reducing recurrence in either study. The explanation for this finding was the amount of red blood cells in the bladder within 30 minutes after TURBT. The red blood cells could inactivate apaziquone, as was observed in previous preclinical intravenous administration of apaziquone.[61]

Safety and tolerability

Apart from evaluation for intravesical use, apaziquone has undergone clinical evaluation when used systemically against a range of tumor types in the past decades, but it has failed to demonstrate activity when administered intravenously. Reasons for the absence of tumor response could be the rapid removal from the blood stream (short half-life time) and poor penetration through avascular tissue.[48] Although these properties are a problem in terms of treating systemic disease, they can be ideal for treating cancers that arise in an anatomically accessible site such as the bladder. Drug delivery is not a problem, as drugs are instilled in the bladder through a catheter. Any drug reaching the blood stream would be rapidly removed,[53,62] making the risk of effects to other tissues low. Furthermore, apaziquone is a bio-reductive drug, so it requires activation by cellular reductase enzymes. As discussed earlier, in the case of apaziquone the enzyme DTD plays a central role in activating the drug. Several tumors have high levels of DTD activity compared with normal tissue, suggesting that selective toxicity against tumor cells may be achieved. In more than 40% of patients suffering from BC, the level of DTD in bladder tumor tissue is higher compared with normal tissue.[63] Another reason to assume systemic toxicity of apaziquone is a minor problem is the fact that systemic absorption through an intact bladder wall into the blood stream is limited because of the molecular weight of 288. Indeed, apaziquone and known metabolites were consistently undetectable by HPLC in the 12 patients of a phase 1 study, 30 and 60 minutes after the start of intravesical instillation with doses ranging from 4 mg to 16 mg in 40 mL,[56] and no hematological changes were noted in the phase 2 study.[60] Finally, apaziquone can be potentiated under acidic extracellular pH (eg, pH 6.0) conditions, but may lose activity in the blood stream because of an increase in extracellular pH to 7.35 to 7.45.

In conclusion, several properties of apaziquone make systemic toxicity unlikely and subsequent intravesical use theoretically safe.

SUMMARY

NMIBC is a common disease with a wide range of oncological outcomes. The optimal treatment has not yet been found, as NMIBC is associated with high rates of recurrence and sometimes progression. Every patient is initially treated with a TURBT, and most patients require adjuvant intravesical instillations of chemotherapeutic or immunotherapeutic drugs. However, as it is common in cancer therapy, instillation therapy is not without toxicity, and even with optimal therapy many patients experience recurrences or even progression.

Progression is a real concern in high-risk patients, especially when they fail standard intravesical therapy with BCG. In these patients failing BCG, the standard therapeutic recommendation is radical surgery, and no conservative treatment is accepted as an alternative.

Nowadays, There are some new promising intravesical therapies/strategies available. Of these newer drugs, gemcitabine seems especially promising, but more studies are needed. CHT shows promising results too, even in patients failing BCG therapy. However, longer follow-up and confirmative randomized data are strongly needed.

Apaziquone is a potent cytotoxic drug. It is activated in the cell with the help of DTD in oxic conditions, or, in its absence, in hypoxia, acting through the redox cycle or DNA breaks. Apaziquone is preferentially active in solid tumor lines. However, it has been ineffective after systemic administration, probably because of its rapid elimination. After intravesical use it is not absorbed from the bladder even, when instilled within 6 hours from TURBT.

Several properties of apaziquone, such as the molecular weight, its metabolic activation, and degradation, make systemic toxicity unlikely; therefore intravesical is considered to be safe.

To date, data of several phase 2 and 2 phase 3 have been published within this field. Although these studies demonstrate the potential of apaziquone, the singular phase 3 trials did not reached their primary endpoint. When their data were pooled, the primary endpoint did reach significance, and a combined post hoc analysis suggested that the installation should be given at least 60 minutes after TURBT. All studies published in the field of apaziquone reported mild adverse effects, comparable to other intravesical drugs, and no systemic adverse effects were noted.

To the authors' best knowledge, there are currently no new trials recruiting. Consulting Clinicaltrials.gov, 1 new phase 3, randomized, multicenter, multiarm, placebo-controlled, double-blind study of apaziquone (NCT02563561) was found. However its recruitment status is "active, not recruiting." Considering the fact that no new trials are recruiting at this moment and current data are insufficient to change any guideline on NMIBC, it seems that the development of apaziquone for NMBIC has stopped. In an FDA Oncological Drugs Advisory Committee (ODAC) meeting of September 14, 2016, the FDA concluded that with the available data apaziquone has not shown substantial evidence of a treatment effect over placebo. This FDA document could be the reason for the study sponsor (Spectrum Pharmaceuticals, Inc.) to focus on other new medicines in its pipelines.

REFERENCES

1. Siegel R, Nalshadham D, Jemal A. Cancer statistics, 2012. CA Cancer J Clin 2012;62:10–29.
2. Sievert KD, Amend B, Nagele U, et al. Economic aspects of bladder cancer: what are the benefits and costs? World J Urol 2009;27:295–300.
3. Ploeg M, Aben KK, Kiemeney LA. The present and future burden of urinary bladder cancer in the world. World J Urol 2009;27:289–93.
4. Babjuk M, Bohle A, Burger M, et al. EAU guidelines on non-muscle-invasive urothelial carcinoma of the bladder: update 2016. Eur Urol 2017;71:447–61.
5. Sylvester RJ, van der Meijden AP, Oosterlinck W, et al. Predicting recurrence and progression in individual patients with stage Ta T1 bladder cancer using EORTC risk tables: a combined analysis of 2596 patients from seven EORTC trials. Eur Urol 2006;49: 466–75 [discussion: 75–7].
6. Fernandez-Gomez J, Madero R, Solsona E, et al. Predicting nonmuscle invasive bladder cancer recurrence and progression in patients treated with *Bacillus Calmette-Guerin*: the CUETO scoring model. J Urol 2009;182:2195–203.
7. Sylvester RJ, Oosterlinck W, van der Meijden AP. A single immediate postoperative instillation of chemotherapy decreases the risk of recurrence in patients with stage Ta T1 bladder cancer: a meta-analysis of published results of randomized clinical trials. J Urol 2004;171:2186–90 [quiz: 435].
8. Brausi M, Collette L, Kurth K, et al. Variability in the recurrence rate at first follow-up cystoscopy after TUR in stage Ta T1 transitional cell carcinoma of

the bladder: a combined analysis of seven EORTC studies. Eur Urol 2002;41:523–31.

9. Guevara A, Salomon L, Allory Y, et al. The role of tumor-free status in repeat resection before intravesical bacillus Calmette-Guerin for high grade Ta, T1 and CIS bladder cancer. J Urol 2010;183:2161–4.

10. Schulze M, Stotz N, Rassweiler J. Retrospective analysis of transurethral resection, second-look resection, and long-term chemo-metaphylaxis for superficial bladder cancer: indications and efficacy of a differentiated approach. J Endourol 2007;21: 1533–41.

11. Schwaibold HE, Sivalingam S, May F, et al. The value of a second transurethral resection for T1 bladder cancer. BJU Int 2006;97:1199–201.

12. Herr HW. The value of a second transurethral resection in evaluating patients with bladder tumors. J Urol 1999;162:74–6.

13. Sylvester RJ, van der MA, Lamm DL. Intravesical Bacillus Calmette-Guerin reduces the risk of progression in patients with superficial bladder cancer: a meta-analysis of the published results of randomized clinical trials. J Urol 2002;168:1964–70.

14. Witjes JA. Management of BCG failures in superficial bladder cancer: a review. Eur Urol 2006;49: 790–7.

15. Pawinski A, Sylvester R, Bouffioux C, et al. A combined analysis of EORTC/MRC randomized clinical trials for the prophylactic treatment of TaT1 bladder cancer. Eortc Genito-Urinary Tract Cancer Cooperative Group and the Medical Research Council Working Party on Superficial Bladder Cancer. Acta Urol Belg 1996;64:27.

16. Witjes JA, Kolli PS. Apaziquone for non-muscle invasive bladder cancer: a critical review. Expert Opin Investig Drugs 2008;17:1085–96.

17. Murta-Nascimento C, Schmitz-Drager BJ, Zeegers MP, et al. Epidemiology of urinary bladder cancer: from tumor development to patient's death. World J Urol 2007;25:285–95.

18. Botteman MF, Pashos CL, Redaelli A, et al. The health economics of bladder cancer: a comprehensive review of the published literature. Pharmacoeconomics 2003;21:1315–30.

19. Blick CG, Nazir SA, Mallett S, et al. Evaluation of diagnostic strategies for bladder cancer using computed tomography (CT) urography, flexible cystoscopy and voided urine cytology: results for 778 patients from a hospital haematuria clinic. BJU Int 2012;110:84–94.

20. Denzinger S, Burger M, Walter B, et al. Clinically relevant reduction in risk of recurrence of superficial bladder cancer using 5-aminolevulinic acid-induced fluorescence diagnosis: 8-year results of prospective randomized study. Urology 2007;69:675–9.

21. Fradet Y, Grossman HB, Gomella L, et al, PC B302/01 Study Group. A comparison of hexaminolevulinate fluorescence cystoscopy and white light cystoscopy for the detection of carcinoma in situ in patients with bladder cancer: a phase III, multicenter study. J Urol 2007;178:68–73 [discussion: 73].

22. Geavlete B, Jecu M, Multescu R, et al. HAL blue-light cystoscopy in high-risk nonmuscle-invasive bladder cancer–re-TURBT recurrence rates in a prospective, randomized study. Urology 2010;76: 664–9.

23. Grossman HB, Gomella L, Fradet Y, et al. A phase III, multicenter comparison of hexaminolevulinate fluorescence cystoscopy and white light cystoscopy for the detection of superficial papillary lesions in patients with bladder cancer. J Urol 2007;178:62–7.

24. Jichlinski P, Guillou L, Karlsen SJ, et al. Hexyl aminolevulinate fluorescence cystoscopy: new diagnostic tool for photodiagnosis of superficial bladder cancer–a multicenter study. J Urol 2003;170:226–9.

25. Jocham D, Witjes F, Wagner S, et al. Improved detection and treatment of bladder cancer using hexaminolevulinate imaging: a prospective, phase III multicenter study. J Urol 2005;174:862–6 [discussion: 6].

26. Schmidbauer J, Witjes F, Schmeller N, et al. Improved detection of urothelial carcinoma in situ with hexaminolevulinate fluorescence cystoscopy. J Urol 2004;171:135–8.

27. Zheng C, Lv Y, Zhong Q, et al. Narrow band imaging diagnosis of bladder cancer: systematic review and meta-analysis. BJU Int 2012;110:E680–7.

28. Cauberg EC, Kloen S, Visser M, et al. Narrow band imaging cystoscopy improves the detection of non-muscle-invasive bladder cancer. Urology 2010;76: 658–63.

29. Herr HW, Donat SM. Reduced bladder tumour recurrence rate associated with narrow-band imaging surveillance cystoscopy. BJU Int 2011;107: 396–8.

30. Mini E, Nobili S, Caciagli B, et al. Cellular pharmacology of gemcitabine. Ann Oncol 2006;17(Suppl 5):v7–12.

31. Kilani RT, Tamimi Y, Karmali S, et al. Selective cytotoxicity of gemcitabine in bladder cancer cell lines. Anticancer Drugs 2002;13:557–66.

32. Laufer M, Ramalingam S, Schoenberg MP, et al. Intravesical gemcitabine therapy for superficial transitional cell carcinoma of the bladder: a phase I and pharmacokinetic study. J Clin Oncol 2003;21: 697–703.

33. Shelley MD, Jones G, Cleves A, et al. Intravesical gemcitabine therapy for non-muscle invasive bladder cancer (NMIBC): a systematic review. BJU Int 2012;109:496–505.

34. Colombo R, Da Pozzo LF, Lev A, et al. Neoadjuvant combined microwave induced local hyperthermia and topical chemotherapy versus chemotherapy

alone for superficial bladder cancer. J Urol 1996;
155:1227–32.

35. Lammers RJ, Witjes JA, Inman BA, et al. The role of a combined regimen with intravesical chemotherapy and hyperthermia in the management of non-muscle-invasive bladder cancer: a systematic review. Eur Urol 2011;60:81–93.

36. Arends TJ, Nativ O, Maffezzini M, et al. Results of a randomised controlled trial comparing intravesical chemohyperthermia with Mitomycin C versus *Bacillus Calmette-Guerin* for adjuvant treatment of patients with intermediate- and high-risk non-muscle-invasive bladder cancer. Eur Urol 2016;69:1046–52.

37. Brausi M, Campo B, Pizzocaro G, et al. Intravesical electromotive administration of drugs for treatment of superficial bladder cancer: a comparative phase II study. Urology 1998;51:506–9.

38. Di Stasi SM, Giannantoni A, Giurioli A, et al. Sequential BCG and electromotive mitomycin versus BCG alone for high-risk superficial bladder cancer: a randomised controlled trial. Lancet Oncol 2006;7: 43–51.

39. Di Stasi SM, Valenti M, Verri C, et al. Electromotive instillation of mitomycin immediately before transurethral resection for patients with primary urothelial non-muscle invasive bladder cancer: a randomised controlled trial. Lancet Oncol 2011;12:871–9.

40. Brake M, Loertzer H, Horsch R, et al. Long-term results of intravesical *Bacillus Calmette-Guerin* therapy for stage T1 superficial bladder cancer. Urology 2000;55:673–8.

41. de Reijke TM, Kurth KH, Sylvester RJ, et al. *Bacillus Calmette-Guerin* versus epirubicin for primary, secondary or concurrent carcinoma in situ of the bladder: results of a European Organization for the Research and Treatment of Cancer–Genito-Urinary Group Phase III Trial (30906). J Urol 2005;173: 405–9.

42. Jakse G, Hall R, Bono A, et al. Intravesical BCG in patients with carcinoma in situ of the urinary bladder: long-term results of EORTC GU Group phase II protocol 30861. Eur Urol 2001;40:144–50.

43. Losa A, Hurle R, Lembo A. Low dose *Bacillus Calmette-Guerin* for carcinoma in situ of the bladder: long-term results. J Urol 2000;163:68–71 [discussion: 2].

44. Yates DR, Brausi MA, Catto JW, et al. Treatment options available for *Bacillus Calmette-Guerin* failure in non-muscle-invasive bladder cancer. Eur Urol 2012; 62:1088–96.

45. van den Bosch S, Alfred Witjes J. Long-term cancer-specific survival in patients with high-risk, non-muscle-invasive bladder cancer and tumour progression: a systematic review. Eur Urol 2011;60: 493–500.

46. Stein JP, Lieskovsky G, Cote R, et al. Radical cystectomy in the treatment of invasive bladder cancer:

long-term results in 1,054 patients. J Clin Oncol 2001;19:666–75.

47. van Lingen AV, Arends TJ, Witjes JA. Expert review: an update in current and developing intravesical therapies for non-muscle-invasive bladder cancer. Expert Rev Anticancer Ther 2013;13:1257–68.

48. Loadman PM, Phillips RM, Lim LE, et al. Pharmacological properties of a new aziridinylbenzoquinone, RH1 (2,5-diaziridinyl-3-(hydroxymethyl)-6-methyl-1,4-benzoquinone), in mice. Biochem Pharmacol 2000;59:831–7.

49. Choudry GA, Stewart PA, Double JA, et al. A novel strategy for NQO1 (NAD(P)H:quinone oxidoreductase, EC 1.6.99.2) mediated therapy of bladder cancer based on the pharmacological properties of EO9. Br J Cancer 2001;85:1137–46.

50. Hoskin PJ, Sibtain A, Daley FM, et al. GLUT1 and CAIX as intrinsic markers of hypoxia in bladder cancer: relationship with vascularity and proliferation as predictors of outcome of ARCON. Br J Cancer 2003; 89:1290–7.

51. Hendriks HR, Pizao PE, Berger DP, et al. EO9: a novel bioreductive alkylating indoloquinone with preferential solid tumour activity and lack of bone marrow toxicity in preclinical models. Eur J Cancer 1993;29A:897–906.

52. van der Heijden AG, Verhaegh G, Jansen CF, et al. Effect of hyperthermia on the cytotoxicity of 4 chemotherapeutic agents currently used for the treatment of transitional cell carcinoma of the bladder: an in vitro study. J Urol 2005;173:1375–80.

53. Workman P, Binger M, Kooistra KL. Pharmacokinetics, distribution, and metabolism of the novel bioreductive alkylating indoloquinone EO9 in rodents. Int J Radiat Oncol Biol Phys 1992;22:713–6.

54. Vainchtein LD, Rosing H, Mirejovsky D, et al. Quantitative analysis of EO9 (apaziquone) and its metabolite EO5a in human plasma by high-performance liquid chromatography under basic conditions coupled to electrospray tandem mass spectrometry. J Mass Spectrom 2006;41:1268–76.

55. Verweij J, Aamdal S, Schellens J, et al. Clinical studies with EO9, a new indoloquinone bioreductive alkylating cytotoxic agent. EORTC Early Clinical Trials Group. Oncol Res 1994;6:519–23.

56. Puri R, Palit V, Loadman PM, et al. Phase I/II pilot study of intravesical apaziquone (EO9) for superficial bladder cancer. J Urol 2006;176:1344–8.

57. Schellens JH, Planting AS, van Acker BA, et al. Phase I and pharmacologic study of the novel indoloquinone bioreductive alkylating cytotoxic drug E09. J Natl Cancer Inst 1994;86:906–12.

58. van der Heijden AG, Moonen PM, Cornel EB, et al. Phase II marker lesion study with intravesical instillation of apaziquone for superficial bladder cancer: toxicity and marker response. J Urol 2006;176: 1349–53 [discussion: 53].

59. Hendricksen K, van der Heijden AG, Cornel EB, et al. Two-year follow-up of the phase II marker lesion study of intravesical apaziquone for patients with non-muscle invasive bladder cancer. World J Urol 2009;27:337–42.

60. Hendricksen K, Cornel EB, de Reijke TM, et al. Phase 2 study of adjuvant intravesical instillations of apaziquone for high risk nonmuscle invasive bladder cancer. J Urol 2012;187:1195–9.

61. Karsh L, Shore N, Soloway M, et al. Double-blind, randomized, placebo-controlled studies evaluating apaziquone (E09, Qapzola) intravesical instillation post transurethral resection of bladder tumors for the treatment of low-risk non-muscle invasive bladder cancer. Bladder Cancer 2018;4: 293–301.

62. McLeod HL, Graham MA, Aamdal S, et al. Phase I pharmacokinetics and limited sampling strategies for the bioreductive alkylating drug EO9. EORTC Early Clinical Trials Group. Eur J Cancer 1996;32A: 1518–22.

63. Li D, Gan Y, Wientjes MG, et al. Distribution of DT-diaphorase and reduced nicotinamide adenine dinucleotide phosphate: cytochrome p450 oxidoreductase in bladder tissues and tumors. J Urol 2001;166:2500–5.

Combination Intravesical Therapy

Nathan A. Brooks, MD, Michael A. O'Donnell, MD*

KEYWORDS

- Salvage therapy • Nonmuscle invasive bladder cancer • BCG failure • Intravesical therapy

KEY POINTS

- Salvage intravesical therapy for nonmuscle invasive bladder cancer remains experimental, and cystectomy should be considered when clinically appropriate.
- Salvage therapy with gemcitabine and docetaxol has the greatest amount of evidence supporting use, is generally well tolerated, and appears efficacious after Bacillus Calmette-Guerin failure.
- This is an exciting time for salvage therapy because there are multiple, ongoing, prospective clinical trials with results expected in the next 2 to 3 years.

INTRODUCTION

Bladder cancer accounts for around 80,000 new cancer diagnoses per year in the United States with 75% of patients presenting with nonmuscle invasive disease. In developed areas, urothelial histology at diagnosis is present in 90% of patients.[1,2] For the subset of patients presenting with high-risk, nonmuscle invasive bladder cancer (NMIBC), intravesical administration of Bacillus Calmette-Guerin (BCG) with maintenance therapy remains the standard of care.[3] BCG administration has largely remained unaltered since its initial description more than 40 years ago and around 40% to 50% of patients will experience recurrence of disease within 5 years of diagnosis with up to 78% of patients experiencing recurrence in the highest-risk groups.[4–6] Recurrence of NMIBC, classified by BCG failure discussed in a previous section, represents a challenging issue to the treating urologist. Clinical guidelines suggest a risk-stratified approach, including a second BCG course, radical cystectomy, or clinical trial enrollment.[3]

Despite these recommendations, utilization of cystectomy remains low, especially among older, more frail patients, those with a lower socioeconomic status, and those in rural communities.[7,8] Practical, salvage alternatives to cystectomy and clinical trial enrollment are therefore of the utmost importance for the patient and the treating urologist, who fail initial BCG administration. Single-agent and device-delivered intravesical therapy have already been discussed. However, as increasing the efficacy of systemic chemotherapy and immunotherapy becomes predicated on multiagent regimens, so might a nuanced approach to intravesical therapy. In this section, multiagent intravesical salvage chemotherapy, immunotherapy, and combined systemic therapy with intravesical therapy are discussed, including a discussion of the mechanisms of action of each (**Table 1**), potential side effects with mitigation strategies, and oncologic outcomes (**Table 2**). Finally, current clinical trials and emerging therapies are discussed (**Table 3**).

Immunotherapy Combinations

Immunotherapy combinations have generally been used to augment the immunogenicity of BCG itself. Therapies have included intravesical and parenteral administration of cytokines, chemokines, and immune checkpoint inhibition.

Department of Urology, The University of Iowa Hospitals and Clinics, 200 Hawkins Drive, Iowa City, IA, USA
* Corresponding author.
E-mail address: michael-odonnell@uiowa.edu

Urol Clin N Am 47 (2020) 83–91
https://doi.org/10.1016/j.ucl.2019.09.010
0094-0143/20/

Table 1
Mechanism of action, common adverse reactions, and doses of intravesical agents administered as part of combination intravesical therapy regimens discussed in this article

Agent	Mechanism of Action	Common Adverse Reactions: Treatment	Dose Administered
IFN	• Inhibit cell proliferation • Enhance immune stimulation • Induce apoptosis	• Fever: antipyretic	50 MU Or 100 MU if used with 1/10th dose BCG
IL-2	• Induce cytotoxic T-cell response	• Fever: antipyretic	22 MU
GMCSF	• Induce cytotoxic T-cell response and enhance function	• Injection site reaction: supportive care	250 μg (subq)
Doxorubicin epirubicin	• Inhibits topoisomerase-II • Direct cell toxicity	• Irritative voiding: antispasmotics	40–50 mg in 50 mL NS
MMC	• Cross-links DNA	• Rash: steroids • Dysuria: analgesics • Bone marrow suppression: hold MMC	20–40 mg in 20–40 mL NS
Gem	• Prevents DNA chain elongation	• Nausea: antiemetic pretreatment	1–2 g in 50 mL NS
Doce	• Inhibits microtube disassembly inhibiting mitosis and cell division	• Generally well tolerated	40 mg (4 mL) in 50 mL NS (final volume 54 mL)

Abbreviations: NS, normal saline; subq, subcutaneously.

Bacillus Calmette-Guerin with interferon

Interferon-α (IFN) has been shown to inhibit cell proliferation, enhance immune stimulation, and lead to cell apoptosis.[9,10] Single-agent IFN demonstrates antitumor prevention activity, although with decreased efficacy compared with BCG.[11] However, synergy between BCG and IFN has been demonstrated with IFN enhancing the BCG immune-mediated response.[12] With this understanding, multiple evaluations of BCG coadministered with IFN have been undertaken, the largest of which enrolled more than 1000 patients in a phase 2, prospective trial of BCG + IFN in patients after prior BCG failure or patients who were BCG naïve.[13,14]

The 467 patients who had failed 1 prior course of BCG received one-third dose BCG with 50 million units (MU) of IFN for a 6-week induction course and then three, 3-week maintenance courses 3, 9, and 15 months after induction completion. Two-year disease-free survival (DFS) in the BCG failure arm was 45% for all patients. Multiple subanalyses from this study have been generated, including the following:

• The efficacy of BCG with IFN significantly declines for each decade older than 50 years old.[15] This is especially evident for patients older than 80, whereby BCG is approximately one-third less effective than in 60- to 70-year-old patients (40% vs 60% 2-year DFS).
• Patients with carcinoma in situ (CIS) and BCG failure within 12 months, refractory disease, or more than 1 course of BCG have a worse response to repeat BCG with IFN.[16]
• BCG failure within 12 months after initial BCG therapy portends a worse prognosis for BCG with IFN.[17]
• BCG with IFN leads to local adverse toxicity during treatment but without effecting long-term quality of life.[18]

A second, prospective, randomized, multicenter study compared BCG ± megadose vitamins with BCG + IFN ± megadose vitamins. All patients in this trial were BCG naïve, and no difference in DFS was determined between treatment arms. However, patients who received BCG with IFN experience more toxicity, including systemic side effects, such as fever and malaise.[19] No

Table 2
Cancer-specific outcomes for the 4 most well-studied, contemporary combination intravesical therapy regimens

Drug Regimen	Complete Response Rate, %	Disease-Free Survival, %	Progression-Free Survival, %	Cystectomy-Free Survival, %	Cancer-Specific Survival, %	Percent Intolerant
1/3 dose BCG + IFN[a,13,14]	79.8	2 y: 45	92.2	96.1	99 at interim analysis	4.8 serious adverse event rate 7.8 intolerance rate
Quadruple immunotherapy[c,24]	65	2 y: 53	92.3 at a median of 11.5 mo	75 at a median of 17.3 mo	2 y: 95 5 y: 82	17.5 delay in treatment schedule, 6 unable to complete induction
Gem + MMC[39–41]	68	2 y: 37–38	Not reported	81	96.3	7.7–15
Gem + Doce[b,44,45]	66	2 y: 24–60	82–94	78–79	2 y: 89–94	11

[a] Six weekly induction course followed by 3 cycles of weekly maintenance there for 3 wk at 3, 9, and 15 mo.
[b] High-grade RFS, 60% ALL grade RFS, 53%.
[c] Includes data from multi-institutional review of 278 patients pending publication.

Table 3
Currently active combination therapy clinical trials for patients with nonmuscle invasive bladder cancer after Bacillus Calmette-Guerin failure

Trial Name	Phase	Agents	Completion Date	Design
Adapt Bladder: NCRN GU16-243 NCT03317158	1/2	1. Durvalumab + BCG 2. Durvalumab + EBRT	9/2021	Randomized, multiarm, crossover
NCT03258593	1	Durvalumab with intravesical oportuzumab monatox	7/2021	Nonrandomized, open-label, single-arm
QUILT-3.032 NCT03022825	2	Intravesical BCG and ALT-803	9/2020	Nonrandomized, open-label, single-arm
NCT01625260	1b/2	Intravenous Gem and intravenous ALT-801	3/2018	Nonrandomized, open-label, single-arm
NCT02015104	1	1. BCG alone 2. BCG with PANVAC	2/2020	Randomized, parallel assignment, open label
NCT02202772[6]	1	1. Gem and cabazitaxel 2. Gem, cisplatin, and cabazitaxel	12/2020	Randomized, open label, multiarm
NCT02792192	1b/2	1. Atezolizumab + BCG 2. Atezolizumab	3/2020	Randomized, parallel assignment, open label

prospective trial had directly compared BCG and BCG with IFN for patients after BCG failure. Given the lack of clear differences in efficacy of BCG and BCG with IFN in BCG-naïve disease and the increased side effects, BCG with IFN likely has limited utility.[20] However, 100 MU IFN with one-tenth dose BCG might show some promise in treating BCG *intolerant* patients.[17]

Quadruple immunotherapy (Bacillus Calmette-Guerin, interferon, interleukin-2, and granulocyte colony stimulating factor)

The success of immunotherapy in NMIBC remains one of the historic triumphs in cancer therapy. Clinically, patients older than 80 experience the largest discrepancy in BCG efficacy.[15] Age-related immune dysfunction has been implicated in this process but remains incompletely understood.[21] Evaluation of the BCG vaccine itself, however, has unveiled that T-cell cytotoxic potential declines with aging.[22] Both granulocyte macrophage colony stimulating factors (granulocyte colony stimulating factor [GMCSF] also sold for injection as sargramostim) and interleukin-2 (IL-2) have been shown to induce and augment a cytotoxic T-cell response.[23]

To circumvent age-related immune response decline, a regimen of 6 weekly intravesical installations of one-third dose BCG, 50 MU IFN, and 22 MU IL-2 in combination with a 250-µg

sargramostim injection (weekly) followed by 3 weekly maintenance treatments at 3, 9, and 15 months has been evaluated retrospectively in 52 patients after BCG failure.[24] The initial response rate to therapy was 65% and DFS was 53% at 2 years. Bladder cancer–specific survival was 82% at 5 years, and 28% of eligible patients underwent cystectomy. Although not statistically significant, DFS was 60% at 2 years in patients older than 80 years old. Notably, 90% of patients experienced a side effect of therapy; 20% of patients required treatment delay, and 6% of patients could not tolerate a full 6-treatment induction course. Quadruple immunotherapy might represent an option for salvage therapy after BCG failure, especially in older adults, although with some tradeoff because patients will likely experience some adverse effects during therapy. Further evaluation needs to be performed.

Bacillus Calmette-Guerin in combination with systemic immunotherapy

The advent of systemic immune checkpoint inhibitor therapy (ICI) and specifically programmed cell death receptor 1 (PD-1) or programmed cell death receptor ligand 1 (PDL-1) blockade for advanced bladder cancer has been met with optimism and early success.[25] Preclinical studies in NMIBC have identified overexpression of PDL-1 on T cells during BCG therapy, shown that blockade of

PDL-1 increases the antitumor response to BCG, and that there is a role for the PD-1/PDL-1 axis in BCG unresponsive disease.[26–29] Mouse models suggest that PDL-1 blockade allows for enhanced local immune-mediated tumor control.[30] Preclinical models and ICI success in advanced disease have provided exciting evidence for the potential efficacy in the NMIBC space. The use of single-agent ICI (pembrolizumab) without concomitant BCG in patients with BCG unresponsive disease has demonstrated a complete response rate of 38.8% and an 80% DFS at 6 months for those with a complete response.[31] Currently, no published results for BCG in combination with systemic immunotherapy for patients after BCG failure are available. However, results of a phase 1 trial (KEYNOTE-676) of BCG with pembrolizumab after BCG failure were recently presented and demonstrated good tolerability and 78% DFS at 5 months.[32] Clinical trials in this area with both ICI monotherapy and combination therapy for BCG and other agents with both atezolizumab (anti-PDL-1) and durvalumab (anti-PDL-1) are ongoing and discussed in the emerging therapy article and **Table 3**.

Chemotherapy Combinations

Historic combination chemotherapy studies
Historic reports on combination intravesical chemotherapy reveal where the urologist has been, so that we may know where we need to go. Most reports are fraught with significant bias, including retrospective studies on small patient populations where classification by BCG failure status and tumor risk are difficult to parse out or simply not provided. The following agents have been studied, and with these limitations in mind, are mentioned for the sake of completeness, but have not gained favor in mainstream practices.

Doxorubicin, mitomycin C, and the addition of cisplatin Doxorubicin is an anthracycline derivative commonly used to treat multiple solid malignancies. The mechanism of action is 2-fold and includes inhibition of topoisomerase-II–mediated DNA repair as well as direct cellular toxicity via free radical generation.[33] Mitomycin C (MMC) is an antitumor antibiotic that acts to cross-link DNA.[34] These 2 agents (20 mg MMC and 40 mg doxorubicin) were compared in the first report of combination intravesical chemotherapy at which time tolerability and efficacy were notably low.[35] As a follow-up to this initial study, a slightly larger cohort of 43 patients (the minority having failed BCG) with carcinoma in situ was evaluated with a progression rate approaching 20%.[36] Likely owing to poor tolerability, efficacy, and significant

disease progression rates, MMC and doxorubicin combination therapy has not been reported in the literature since 1994. A regimen of MMC, doxorubicin, and intravesical cisplatin was reported for BCG-naïve patients in comparison to BCG alone with promising results, although the addition of intravesical cisplatin resulted in severe, debilitating lower urinary tract symptoms for several patients.[37] This regimen has not been evaluated further.

Epirubicin and interferon-alpha A prospective, randomized trial that evaluated instillation of epirubicin with IFN-α compared with BCG in patients naïve to intravesical therapy demonstrated superiority of BCG for preventing recurrence without a difference in adverse events or progression.[38,39] Further evaluation of this regimen in the salvage setting has not been performed.

Gemcitabine, cabazitaxel, and cisplatin First reported in a phase 1 trial in 2017 in 9 BCG-refractory patients, gemcitabine, cabazitaxel, and cisplatin (GCP) intravesical therapy was noted to be well tolerated and associated with a 78% complete response rate.[40] This trial was expanded to 18 BCG-unresponsive in 2019. Results of a phase 1 study redemonstrated tolerability as well as a complete response rate of 94% and a DFS of 78% at 9.5 months.[41] Results with GCP are promising; however, results have only been presented thus far in abstract form.

Modern combination chemotherapy studies
The following studies represent the more well-studied combination intravesical chemotherapy regimens. Studies are generally hampered by the retrospective nature of their results but are bolstered, if only slightly, through larger, more well-defined patient cohorts. Recommended administration regimen, side effects, and outcomes are reported in **Tables 1** and **2**.

Gemcitabine and mitomycin C Gemcitabine (Gem) is a deoxynucleotide analogue, which prevents DNA chain elongation during DNA synthesis.[42] First reported in 2006, the combination of sequentially administered salvage Gem and MMC showed promising results (20-month median DFS) in 27 patients after BCG failure.[43] Further evaluation of this regimen as salvage therapy after BCG therapy has been performed at multiple institutions. Two-year DFS was reported at 37% and 38%; progression occurred in 3.7% of patients, and 19% of patients underwent radical cystectomy. The regimen was generally well tolerated with most adverse events related to the MMC component or Gem-induced nausea.[44,45]

Nausea may be treated with prophylactic ondansetron.

Administration Administration order for these agents is thought to be important. Patients should be pretreated with an oral urinary alkalization agent (such as 1300 mg sodium bicarbonate the night before and the morning of installation). Gem does not generally directly irritate the bladder; however, its solution is very acidic (pH ~2.6), whereby MMC is inactivated under acidic conditions and does irritate the bladder. Patients receive 6 weekly intravesical installations for induction, which includes administration of the following:

- 1 g Gem in 50 mL normal saline (dwell time: 90 minutes)
- The bladder is drained without rinsing
- Instill 40 mg MMC diluted in 20 mL sterile saline (dwell time 90 minutes)

Monthly maintenance administrations are generally given for 1 to 2 years or until recurrence.

Gemcitabine and docetaxol Docetaxol (Doce) inhibits microtube disassembly inhibiting mitosis and cell division.[46] Recent preclinical work has demonstrated that Gem acts as an exfoliant for urothelial cells increasing the cellular penetration efficacy of Doce.[47] Gem/Doce thus represents one of the most promising new intravesical salvage therapy regimens. The efficacy of salvage Gem/Doce has been evaluated in 2 retrospective series. One- and 2-year DFS ranged from 42% to 54% and 27% to 37%, respectively. Up to 10% of patients experienced disease progression to muscle invasive disease.[48,49] Preliminary results from a multi-institutional analysis of 278 patients receiving salvage Gem/Doce demonstrated that the regimen was very well tolerated with less than 5% of patients discontinuing therapy, a 60% high-grade recurrence free survival at 2 years, 6% progression rate to muscle invasive disease, 94% 2-year cancer-specific survival, and 15% cystectomy rate (Michael A. O'Donnell, 2019, unpublished data). These promising results will likely lead to a multi-institutional, prospective evaluation of Gem/Doce in the salvage setting.

Administration Patients should be pretreated with an oral urinary alkalization agent (such as 1300 mg sodium bicarbonate the night before and the morning of installation). Gem can induce nausea, and pretreatment with ondansetron can be beneficial. Neither Gem nor Doce irritates the bladder. Patients receive 6 weekly intravesical installations for induction, which includes administration of the following:

- 1 g Gem in 50 mL normal saline (dwell time: 90 minutes)
- The bladder is drained without rinsing
- 40 mg of Doce instilled, diluted in 50 mL sterile saline (dwell time: 90–120 minutes)

Monthly maintenance administrations are generally given for 1 to 2 years or until recurrence.

Current clinical trials and emerging therapies
Given the tangible need for better, bladder-sparing treatment options after BCG failure, multiple, combination therapy regimens continue to emerge. Guidance from the Food and Drug Administration (FDA) (updated in 2018) regarding trial design includes documenting an initial complete response rate whereby the lower bound of the 95% confidence interval rules out a nonmeaningful response at 3 months for CIS and a clinically meaningful, durable DFS.[50] Trials are generally single-arm, phase 2 clinical trials. Current clinical trials evaluating combination therapy are reviewed in **Table 3**.

Novel agents in these clinical trials include the following:

- Oportuzumab monatox, an antibody to the Epithelial Cell Adhesion Molecule, fused to a bacterial toxin, which has shown initial promise when administered alone for NMIBC after BCG failure.[51]
- ALT-803, an IL-15 superagonist, which has been shown to be an effective and well-tolerated intravesical additive to BCG treatment in BCG-naïve patients.[52]
- ALT-801, an IL-2 agonist, which has shown promise in combination with systemic ICI for metastatic bladder cancer.[53]
- PANVAC pox virus vaccine therapy targeting 2 common overexpressed cancer genes: carcinoembryonic antigen and epithelial mucin 1.[54]

Multiple additional clinic trials for single-agent or device-delivered therapy are also ongoing.[55,56] Most trial results are expected by 2021, making this an exciting time for growth in this field for both the urologist and patient.

SUMMARY

The management of the 30% to 40% of patients with recurrent high-risk, NMIBC after initial definitive intravesical therapy remains a quagmire: burdened by the weight of poor-quality, muddied evidence admixed with time-consuming, often morbid, and sometimes effective therapy.

Although clinical guidelines suggest radical extirpative therapy, many patients are unfit, and urologists remain unwilling to perform this, for good reason. Data supporting the use of cystectomy are retrospective in nature with disease progressing in 1% to 70% of patients, although generally only after a surgery delay of 1 to 2 years.[6,57] Thus, there is very likely a window whereby salvage therapy might play a role in disease treatment and bladder preservation. Pragmatically, enrollment of patients in a trial whereby they receive radical cystectomy versus intravesical therapy in this setting is unlikely to accrue given the major difference in therapies. Having recognized the aforementioned limitations, the FDA has now approved guidance for clinical trial design in this setting, and, going forward, many single- and combination-agent clinical trials promise results reporting by 2021.

Until such time, the urologist must make every effort to guide patients through the milieu of treatment options. Combination agent intravesical therapy presents an excitingly efficacious avenue. Combinations of BCG with IFN have so far not demonstrated a benefit for BCG unresponsive patients, but may be useful, allowing for dose reduction to one-tenth dose BCG for patients previously BCG intolerant. Likewise, quadruple immunotherapy with one-third dose BCG may provide some benefit, possibly for patients with age-related immune dysfunction, however, with an increased incidence of side effects and therapy discontinuation than BCG alone. Historic combination chemotherapy regimens as discussed above were never explored in large patient populations. However, combination therapy with Gem/MMC and Gem/Doce has been reviewed in the largest series of patients at multiple institutions. Results from a large, multi-institutional analysis of Gem/Doce suggest that 2-year, high-risk DFS occurs in 60% of patients with only a 6% progression rate, and less than a 5% discontinuation rate owing to side effects, thus making Gem/Doce the most well studied, well tolerated, and efficacious combination chemotherapy regimen in this patient population. One barrier to Gem/Doce and Gem/MMC instillations is the requirement of a fume hood at the practice site for therapy mixing. However, a fume hood will soon be required for mixing of BCG, which will necessitate this expense if intravesical therapy is a part of the practice.

To date, combination intravesical therapy, especially with Gem/Doce, represents an available promising treatment of salvage therapy in patients with high-risk NMIBC who are unfit or unwilling to undergo cystectomy. These therapy alternatives remain outside the standard of care and do not replace definitive surgical cure. Prior to initiating therapy, this should be discussed with the patient. Growth in this field of study is currently taking off with several exciting clinical trial results expected over the next several years. It is the authors' hope that evidence-based alternatives to cystectomy and a better understanding of targeting therapy to specific patients and tumors will begin to change the treatment paradigm in this challenging and complex patient population.

DISCLOSURE STATEMENT

This work was partially supported by the John and Carol Walter Family Foundation.

REFERENCES

1. Sanli O, Dobruch J, Knowles MA, et al. Bladder cancer. Nat Rev Dis Primers 2017;3:17022.
2. Burger M, Catto JWF, Dalbagni G, et al. Epidemiology and risk factors of urothelial bladder cancer. Eur Urol 2013;63(2):234–41.
3. Chang SS, Boorjian SA, Chou R, et al. Diagnosis and treatment of non-muscle invasive bladder cancer: AUA/SUO guideline. J Urol 2016;196(4):1021–9.
4. Oddens J, Brausi M, Sylvester R, et al. Final results of an EORTC-GU cancers group randomized study of maintenance bacillus Calmette-Guerin in intermediate- and high-risk Ta, T1 papillary carcinoma of the urinary bladder: one-third dose versus full dose and 1 year versus 3 years of maintenance. Eur Urol 2013;63(3):462–72.
5. Lamm DL, Blumenstein BA, Crissman JD, et al. Maintenance bacillus Calmette-Guerin immunotherapy for recurrent TA, T1 and carcinoma in situ transitional cell carcinoma of the bladder: a randomized Southwest Oncology Group Study. J Urol 2000; 163(4):1124–9.
6. Sylvester RJ, van der Meijden AP, Oosterlinck W, et al. Predicting recurrence and progression in individual patients with stage Ta T1 bladder cancer using EORTC risk tables: a combined analysis of 2596 patients from seven EORTC trials. Eur Urol 2006; 49(3):466–77.
7. Williams SB, Hudgins HK, Ray-Zack MD, et al. Systematic review of factors associated with the utilization of radical cystectomy for bladder cancer. Eur Urol Oncol 2019;2(2):119–25.
8. Jacobs BL, Montgomery JS, Zhang Y, et al. Disparities in bladder cancer. Urol Oncol Semin Original Invest 2012;30(1):81–8.
9. Papageorgiou A, Dinney CPN, McConkey DJ. Interferon-α induces TRAIL expression and cell death via

an IRF-1-dependent mechanism in human bladder cancer cells. Cancer Biol Ther 2007;6(6):872–9.

10. Pfeffer LM, Dinarello CA, Herberman RB, et al. Biological properties of recombinant α-interferons: 40th anniversary of the discovery of interferons. Cancer Res 1998;58(12):2489–99.

11. Jimenez-Cruz JF, Vera-Donoso CD, Leiva O, et al. Intravesical immunoprophylaxis in recurrent superficial bladder cancer (stage T1): multicenter trial comparing bacille Calmette-Guérin and interferon-alpha. Urology 1997;50(4):529–35.

12. Luo Y, Chen X, Downs TM, et al. IFN-α 2B enhances Th1 cytokine responses in bladder cancer patients receiving Mycobacterium bovis bacillus Calmette-Guerin immunotherapy. J Immunol 1999;162(4): 2399–405.

13. Joudi FN, Smith BJ, O'Donnell MA. Final results from a national multicenter phase II trial of combination bacillus Calmette-Guérin plus interferon α-2B for reducing recurrence of superficial bladder cancer. Urol Oncol Semin Original Invest 2006;24(4):344–8.

14. O'Donnell Michael A, Lilli K, Leopold C. Interim results from a national,multicenter phase II trial of combination BCG plus IFN alpha 2B for superficial bladder cancer. J Urol 2004;172(3):888–93.

15. Joudi FN, Smith BJ, O'Donnell MA, et al. The impact of age on the response of patients with superficial bladder cancer to intravesical immunotherapy. J Urol 2006;175(5):1634–40.

16. Gallagher BL, Joudi FN, Maymí JL, et al. Impact of previous bacille Calmette-Guérin failure pattern on subsequent response to bacille Calmette-Guérin plus interferon intravesical therapy. Urology 2008; 71(2):297–301.

17. Rosevear HM, Lightfoot AJ, Birusingh KK, et al. Factors affecting response to bacillus Calmette-Guérin plus interferon for urothelial carcinoma in situ. J Urol 2011;186(3):817–23.

18. Steinberg RL, Thomas LJ, Mott SL, et al. Multiperspective tolerance evaluation of bacillus Calmette-Guerin with interferon in the treatment of non-muscle invasive bladder cancer. Bladder Cancer 2019;5(1):39–49.

19. Nepple KG, Lightfoot AJ, Rosevear HM, et al. Bacillus Calmette-Guérin with or without interferon α-2b and megadose versus recommended daily allowance vitamins during induction and maintenance intravesical treatment of nonmuscle invasive bladder cancer. J Urol 2010;184(5):1915–9.

20. Shepherd AR, Shepherd E, Brook NR. Intravesical bacillus Calmette-Guérin with interferon-alpha versus intravesical bacillus Calmette-Guérin for treating non-muscle-invasive bladder cancer. Cochrane Database Syst Rev 2017;(3):CD012112.

21. Hurez V, Padrón ÁS, Svatek RS, et al. Considerations for successful cancer immunotherapy in aged hosts. Clin Exp Immunol 2017;187(1):53–63.

22. Nandakumar S, Kannanganat S, Posey JE, et al. Attrition of T-cell functions and simultaneous up-regulation of inhibitory markers correspond with the waning of BCG-induced protection against tuberculosis in mice. PLoS One 2014;9(11): e113951.

23. Luo Y, Chen X, O'Donnell MA. Role of Th1 and Th2 cytokines in BCG-induced IFN-γ production: cytokine promotion and simulation of BCG effect. Cytokine 2003;21(1):17–26.

24. Steinberg RL, Nepple KG, Velaer KN, et al. Quadruple immunotherapy of bacillus Calmette-Guérin, interferon, interleukin-2, and granulocyte-macrophage colony-stimulating factor as salvage therapy for non-muscle-invasive bladder cancer. Urol Oncol Semin Original Invest 2017;35(12):670. e7-14.

25. Rijnders M, de Wit R, Boormans JL, et al. Systematic review of immune checkpoint inhibition in urological cancers. Eur Urol 2017;72(3):411–23.

26. Wang Y, Liu J, Yang X, et al. Bacillus Calmette–Guérin and anti-PD-l1 combination therapy boosts immune response against bladder cancer. Onco targets Ther 2018;11:2891.

27. Inman BA, Sebo TJ, Frigola X, et al. PD-L1 (B7-H1) expression by urothelial carcinoma of the bladder and BCG-induced granulomata. Cancer 2007; 109(8):1499–505.

28. Chevalier MF, Schneider AK, Cesson V, et al. Conventional and PD-L1-expressing regulatory T cells are enriched during BCG therapy and may limit its efficacy. Eur Urol 2018;74(5):540–4.

29. Mukherjee N, Svatek R. Cancer immune therapy: prognostic significance and implications for therapy of PD-1 in BCG-relapsing bladder cancer. Ann Surg Oncol 2018;25(9):2498–9.

30. Vandeveer AJ, Fallon JK, Tighe R, et al. Systemic immunotherapy of non-muscle invasive mouse bladder cancer with avelumab, an anti-PD-L1 immune checkpoint inhibitor. Cancer Immunol Res 2016;4(5):452–62.

31. Kulkarini GS, Wit RD, Balar AV, et al. MP43-01: phase 2 keynote-057 study: pembrolizumab for patients with high-risk non-muscle invasive bladder cancer unresponsive to bacillus Calmette-Guerin. J Urol 2019;201(Supplement 4):e616.

32. Alanee S, El-Zawahry A, McVary K, et al. MP43-09: phase I trial of intravesical bacillus Calmette-Guérin combined with intravenous pembrolizumab in high grade nonmuscle invasive bladder cancer. J Urol 2019;201(Supplement 4):e620–1.

33. Thorn CF, Oshiro C, Marsh S, et al. Doxorubicin pathways: pharmacodynamics and adverse effects. Pharmacogenetics·Genomics 2011;21(7):440.

34. Verweij J, Pinedo HM. Mitomycin C: mechanism of action, usefulness and limitations. Anticancer Drugs 1990;1(1):5–13.

35. Fukui I, Sekine H, Kihara K, et al. Intravesical combination chemotherapy with mitomycin C and doxorubicin for carcinoma in situ of the bladder. J Urol 1989;141(3 Part 1):531–3.

36. Sekine H, Fukui I, Yamada T, et al. Intravesical mitomycin C and doxorubicin sequential therapy for carcinoma in situ of the bladder: a longer followup result. J Urol 1994;151(1):27–30.

37. Chen C-H, Yang H-J, Shun C-T, et al. A cocktail regimen of intravesical mitomycin-C, doxorubicin, and cisplatin (MDP) for non-muscle-invasive bladder cancer. Urol Oncol Semin Original Invest 2012;30(4):421–7.

38. Duchek M, Johansson R, Jahnson S, et al. Bacillus Calmette-Guerin is superior to a combination of epirubicin and interferon-a2b in the intravesical treatment of patients with stage T1 urinary bladder cancer. A prospective, randomized, Nordic study. Eur Urol 2010;57(1):25–31.

39. Marttila T, Järvinen R, Liukkonen T, et al. Intravesical bacillus Calmette-Guérin versus combination of epirubicin and interferon-α2a in reducing recurrence of non–muscle-invasive bladder carcinoma: FinnBladder-6 study. Eur Urol 2016;70(2):341–7.

40. DeCastro G, Sui W, Pak J, et al. MP15-13 a phase I trial for the use of intravesical cabazitaxel, gemcitabine, and cisplatin (CGC) in the treatment of BCG-refractory non-muscle invasive urothelial carcinoma of the bladder. J Urol 2017;197(4S):e175–6.

41. DeCastro GJ, Anderson C, Pak J, et al. MP43-14;a phase 1 trial of intravesical cabazitaxel, gemcitabine, and cisplatin (CGC) for the treatment of non-muscle invasive BCG unresponsive urothelial carcinoma of the bladder. J Urol 2019;201(Supplement 4):e623.

42. Plunkett W, Huang P, Xu Y-Z, et al. Gemcitabine: metabolism, mechanisms of action, and self-potentiation. Seminars in oncology 1995;22(4S):3–10.

43. Maymi Jose L, Saltsgaver N, O'Donnell MA. 840: Intravesical sequential gemcitabine-mitomycin chemotherapy as salvage treatment for patients with refractory superficial bladder cancer. J Urol 2006;175(4S):271.

44. Cockerill PA, Knoedler JJ, Frank I, et al. Intravesical gemcitabine in combination with mitomycin C as salvage treatment in recurrent non-muscle-invasive bladder cancer. BJU Int 2016;117(3):456–62.

45. Lightfoot AJ, Breyer BN, Rosevear HM, et al. Multi-institutional analysis of sequential intravesical gemcitabine and mitomycin C chemotherapy for non–muscle invasive bladder cancer. Urologic Oncology: Seminars and Original Investigations 2014;32(1):35.e15.

46. Herbst RS, Khuri FR. Mode of action of docetaxel–a basis for combination with novel anticancer agents. Cancer Treat Rev 2003;29(5):407–15.

47. Pandey R, Jackson JK, Liggins R, et al. Enhanced taxane uptake into bladder tissues following co-administration with either mitomycin C, doxorubicin or gemcitabine: association to exfoliation processes. BJU Int 2018;122(5):898–908.

48. Milbar N, Kates M, Chappidi MR, et al. Oncological outcomes of intravesical gemcitabine and docetaxel for select patients with high grade recurrent NMIBC. J Clin Oncol 2017;35(15_suppl):4546.

49. Steinberg RL, Thomas LJ, O'Donnell MA, et al. Sequential intravesical gemcitabine and docetaxel for the salvage treatment of non-muscle invasive bladder cancer. Bladder Cancer 2015;1(1):65–72.

50. Jarow JP, Lerner SP, Kluetz PG, et al. Clinical trial design for the development of new therapies for nonmuscle-invasive bladder cancer: report of a Food and Drug Administration and American Urological Association public workshop. Urology 2014;83(2):262–5.

51. Dickstein R, Wu N, Cowan B, et al. LBA27 phase 3 study of vicinium in BCG-unresponsive non-muscle invasive bladder cancer: initial results. J Urol 2018;199(4, Supplement):e1167.

52. Rosser CJ, Nix J, Ferguson L, et al. Phase Ib trial of ALT-803, an IL-15 superagonist, plus BCG for the treatment of BCG-naïve patients with non-muscle-invasive bladder cancer. J Clin Oncol 2018;36(6_suppl):510.

53. Gupta S, Gill D, Poole A, et al. Systemic immunotherapy for urothelial cancer: current trends and future directions. Cancer 2017;9(2):15.

54. Brancato SJ, Stamatakis L, Apolo AB, et al. A randomized, prospective, phase II study to determine the efficacy of BCG given in combination with PANVAC versus BCG alone in adults with high grade non-muscle invasive bladder cancer who failed at least one induction course of BCG. J Clin Oncol 2014;32(15_suppl):TPS4590.

55. Nykopp TK, da Costa JB, Mannas M, et al. Current clinical trials in non-muscle invasive bladder cancer. Curr Urol Rep 2018;19(12):101.

56. DeCastro GJ, Sui W, Pak JS, et al. A phase I trial for the use of intravesical cabazitaxel, gemcitabine, and cisplatin (CGC) in the treatment of BCG-refractory nonmuscle invasive urothelial carcinoma of the bladder. J Clin Oncol 2017;35(6_suppl):313.

57. Brooks NA, O'Donnell MA. Treatment options in non-muscle-invasive bladder cancer after BCG failure. Indian J Urol 2015;31(4):312–9.

Intravesical Gene Therapy

Vikram M. Narayan, MD, Colin P.N. Dinney, MD*

KEYWORDS

- Intravesical gene therapy • Bladder cancer • BCG-unresponsive • Interferon-alpha
- Immunogene therapy

KEY POINTS

- Non–muscle-invasive bladder cancer is usually treated with transurethral resection followed by intravesical bacillus Calmette-Guerin.
- For patients who develop bacillus Calmette-Guerin-unresponsive disease but cannot tolerate surgery, there are few effective salvage intravesical options, with valrubicin only conferring a 10% complete response.
- Gene therapy is the delivery of nucleic acid into a host's cell to produce a therapeutic effect; intravesical gene therapy can modulate the host's immune response and generate an antitumor response.
- Adenoviral vectors can deliver gene therapy into normal and tumor cells, and recombinant Ad-IFN-α2b has demonstrated encouraging results in phase I and phase II settings.
- Combination of other agents with intravesical gene therapy constructs and the identification of novel biomarkers to aid in treatment selection remains an area of ongoing research.

INTRODUCTION AND BACKGROUND

Non–muscle-invasive bladder cancer (NMIBC) is a challenging disease to treat. These patients are typically treated with transurethral resection followed in most cases by intravesical therapy, to decrease the risk of disease recurrence and progression while maintaining a functional bladder.[1] Unfortunately, most patients remain at risk for tumor recurrence and nearly a third progress to muscle-invasive disease.[2] Additional intravesical options are urgently needed to mitigate the risk of progression to secondary muscle-invasive bladder cancer and early cystectomy.

MANAGING NON–MUSCLE-INVASIVE BLADDER CANCER WITH BACILLUS CALMETTE-GUERIN

Bacillus Calmette-Guerin (BCG) was initially developed as a vaccine for tuberculosis, and it is a live attenuated drug derived from *Mycobacterium bovis*. The use of BCG for the treatment of cancer can be traced back to the observations of Pearl[3] in 1929, when patients with a diagnosis of tuberculosis were noted to have lower rates of cancer at the time of their autopsies. In 1976, Morales and colleagues[4] published a landmark study describing the first use of BCG to treat bladder cancer intravesically. The intravesical introduction

Disclosures: V.M. Narayan: declares no conflicts of interest. C.P.N. Dinney: Independent Chairman of the Adstiladrin Phase III trial for FKD Therapies Oy, and research for NCI, and the University of Eastern Finland, Faculty of Health Sciences (UEHFS).
Funding: The University of Texas MD Anderson Cancer Center SPORE in Genitourinary Cancer P50CA091846, NIH/NCI under P30CA016672.
University of Texas MD Anderson Cancer Center, 1515 Holcombe Boulevard, Unit 1373, Houston, TX 77030, USA
* Corresponding author.
E-mail address: cdinney@mdanderson.org
Twitter: @VikramNarayan (V.M.N.)

urologic.theclinics.com

of BCG causes an infection of urothelial and tumor cells through a fibronectin-mediated process.[5] This, in turn, promotes a local immune response facilitated by granulocytes, macrophages, and T-helper cells. Antitumor responses result partly from the antigen-processing functions of these phagocytic cells. Several cytokines, including tumor necrosis factor-α, interferon (IFN), and IL-1, IL-2, IL-6, IL-8, IL-10, IL-12, and IL-17 participate in the immune stimulation process as demonstrated by post-BCG urine analysis.[6,7] More recently, the role of autophagy in generating an epigenetic reprogramming of monocytes ("trained immunity") has also been implicated in the mechanism of generating an intravesical BCG-stimulated host response.[8]

The antitumor activity of BCG is therefore derived from both the adaptive and innate immune systems of the patient. Intravesical administration stimulates an immune response via cytokine release, including IL-2, tumor necrosis factor-α, IFN-γ, and IL-12 among others. CD4$^+$ T cells and CD8$^+$ cytotoxic T cells produce much of the adaptive antitumor response, whereas the innate immune system is driven by natural killer cells, neutrophils, dendritic cells, and macrophages.

In clinical trials, intravesical BCG has demonstrated initial complete response (CR) rates that vary between 55% and 65% for papillary tumors and 70% to 75% for carcinoma in situ (CIS).[9,10] Despite the benefits demonstrated in both decreased progression and recurrence rates, more than one-third of patients fail BCG therapy and an additional 40% of initial responders are found to have relapsed within 5 years of treatment.[11]

UNDERSTANDING THE GENOMICS OF NON–MUSCLE-INVASIVE BLADDER CANCER

Advances in whole genome sequencing technology have vastly improved our insights into the complexity and heterogeneity of bladder cancer. In particular, parallel efforts to comprehensively characterize the molecular composition of muscle-invasive disease have revealed that muscle-invasive bladder cancer can be broadly grouped into basal and luminal subtypes that are similar to those found in breast cancer, with distinct clinical features.[12–14] Efforts to similarly characterize NMIBC have also been undertaken, with mutations identified in the TERT promoter,[15] FGFR3,[16–18] PIK3CA,[19] and STAG2.[20] Hurst and colleagues[21] described 2 genomic subtypes for stage Ta tumors; one group (named genomic subtype 1) was characterized by no detectable copy-number alterations, and the second group (genomic subtype 2) was defined by a loss of chromosome 9q.

GENE THERAPY DEFINITIONS

Gene therapy refers to the delivery of nucleic acid into a host's cell to produce a therapeutic effect.[22] The US Food and Drug Administration definition of gene therapy notes that they include products that "mediate their effects by transcription and/or translation of transferred genetic material and/or by integrating into the host genome . . . administered as nucleic acids, viruses, or genetically engineered microorganisms."[23] Gene therapy can thus either target tumor cells directly to repair mutated tumor suppressor functions, or it can modulate the host's immune response to generate an antitumor response (so-called immunogene therapy).[24] Early gene therapy studies attempted to replace a defective gene with a normal copy of the affected gene and focused on treatment of genetically inherited diseases such as cystic fibrosis or muscular dystrophy.[25]

Most research efforts today focus on using gene therapy to treat human malignancies. The most common gene transfer vectors used in clinical trials include adenoviral, retroviral, and naked plasmid vectors, and there are currently more than 1800 approved gene therapy clinical trials worldwide.[23]

EARLY GENE THERAPY EFFORTS IN BLADDER CANCER

Initial gene therapy efforts focused on ways to restore the normal function of tumor suppressor genes in urothelial cell carcinoma. Specifically, p53 and retinoblastoma, two tumor suppressor genes that are known to be mutated in 40% to 60% of bladder cancers and confer a worse prognosis, were targeted using replication-deficient adenoviral vectors by our group at the MD Anderson Cancer Center.[26–28] Both p53 and retinoblastoma are involved in the regulation of normal cell cycle functions as well as programmed cell death. Human epithelial cells, including urothelial cell carcinoma cells, are uniquely susceptible to an adenoviral infection owing to the presence of the coxsackie/adenovirus receptor.[29] In preclinical studies, the in vivo transfer of wild-type human p53 into urothelial cancer cells was shown to inhibit the growth of these cells, putatively through the completion of a previously defective apoptotic pathway.[28] Replication-deficient adenoviral vectors work by infecting cells during the cell cycle but cannot replicate in vivo.[29] Transferred genes can thus persist within the infected cell for about 2 weeks.[30]

Intravesical instillation of adenoviral vectors was initially carried out using a reporter gene to verify successful viral-mediated transfection within animal models. Morris and colleagues[31] intravesically delivered an adenoviral vector containing β-galactosidase into the bladders of rats, subsequently assessing the efficiency of gene transfer and the impact of this gene therapy on the histology of the affected cells. They found that not only was the adenovirus-mediated gene transfer effective, but also that the bladder architecture was histologically indistinguishable from normal controls without any evidence of cystitis or systemic spread of the infection (as determined by polymerase chain reaction-based assessments for the gene product within the kidneys, heart, and lung extracts from the intravesically treated rats).[31]

Kuball and colleagues[32] conducted an open-label, single-center phase I study evaluating both intratumoral injection as well as intravesical instillation of recombinant-adenovirus/p53 (SCH 58500), which encoded the wild-type p53 human cDNA. This study was conducted in patients with invasive bladder cancer who were scheduled for radical cystectomy, so as to allow for the evaluation of postcystectomy tissue sampling to understand treatment response. The agent was delivered intravesically through a catheter in 2 sequential administrations, with a dwell time of 60 minutes for each instillation. Before instillation, the bladders were primed with a transduction-enhancing agent called Big CHAP.[33] Eight patients ultimately received intravesical instillation and underwent cystectomy with tissue available for analysis. Key findings included grades 2 and 3 urethral and vesical burning reported by patients during instillation and dwell time within the bladder, but no systemic toxicities were observed. Detectable p53 transgene expression was identified in 7 of 8 bladder tumors that had received an intravesical instillation. Although this study was not designed to establish clinical efficacy, it represented a novel proof-of-concept for the safety and biologic feasibility of intravesical gene therapy in humans with bladder cancer.[32]

Our group at MD Anderson also conducted a phase I, dose-escalation study using Ad5CMV-p53, administered intravesically to cystectomy-ineligible patients with measurable, locally advanced urothelial cell carcinoma of the bladder.[34] In this study, wild-type human p53 cDNA was combined with a cytomegalovirus promoter and a replication-defective adenoviral vector. Instillations were performed daily through a Foley catheter at different doses and patients were monitored for adverse events for at least 12 months. Thirteen patients were treated (10 with prior muscle-invasive bladder cancer and 3 with extensive recurrent superficial disease after BCG).[34] None of the patients in this trial experienced dose-limiting toxicity, and the most common complaint was bladder spasms, observed most often in the higher dose levels. Two out of 7 patients with assessable tissue samples showed vector-specific p53 expression after treatment, and both had received the higher dosing schedule.[34] Overall, the low efficiency of gene transfer was in part attributed to the protective glycosoaminoglycan (GAG) layer of the bladder mucosa, as well potentially lower levels of coxsackie/adenovirus receptor expression within the patients treated. In addition, detecting p53 staining was made more challenging by the fact that most patients in the study had abnormally high p53 staining at baseline, likely owing to the advanced disease state of the included study population. Nevertheless, the study provided confidence as to the general safety of intravesical gene therapy and highlighted some important limitations that future trials would need to consider.

PRIMING THE BLADDER FOR INTRAVESICAL GENE THERAPY

The urothelium of the bladder is a complex, multilayer surface that is tasked with providing a barrier from pathogens and urinary waste products.[35] The superficial part of surface is also known as the GAG layer and is composed of a hydrophilic, polyanionic barrier of glycoproteins and proteoglycans. The main components of the GAG layer include chondroitin sulfate and hyaluronic acid, and these in part work to provide protection against the unwanted internalization of ions, solutes, water, and urinary bacteria that may be present in excreted urine.[35] Dysfunction of the GAG layer has been implicated in interstitial cystitis and the development of chronic pelvic pain syndrome.[35]

Successful intravesical gene therapy requires a means to permeate the GAG layer such that the underlying urothelium can be accessed for efficient viral transduction. As noted elsewhere in this article, the nonionic detergent Big CHAP was an early transduction-promoting agent used in initial intravesical adenoviral vector clinical studies, described first by Connor and colleagues.[33] Further investigation of this agent led to the discovery of Syn3, a polyamide compound demonstrated to improve intravesical gene delivery.[36] This compound would prove to be essential in overcoming the intravesical gene transduction limitations encountered in previous clinical trials.

IMMUNOGENE THERAPY USING INTERFERON

Immunogene therapy refers to the delivery of genetic material for the purpose of modulating a host immune response. In immunogene therapy, tumor-induced immunosuppression can be altered, and antigen-specific antitumor responses can be stimulated. Therapies such as high-dose IL-2 have been used effectively in treating renal cell carcinoma, albeit with significant systemic adverse events. IFN-α belongs to the family of cytokine proteins and works to pleiotropically impede tumor cell growth. IFN-α has been demonstrated to augment the response of T helper type 1 immune responses when combined with BCG, and as such its use as combination therapy with BCG has been explored in several trials. In a national multi-institutional phase II trial evaluate the combination of IFN-α and BCG in patients with non–muscle-invasive disease, 59% of BCG-naïve and 45% of prior BCG-unresponsive patients remained disease free at 24-month.[37] A hypothetical way to potentiate the immunogene effect of IFN-α may be to deliver it within a gene therapy/adenoviral construct, ideally increasing the transfection rate of IFN-α into urothelial cells and stimulating an immune response by virtue of the adenovirus vehicle itself (**Fig. 1**). Unlike the delivery of systemic cytokines such as IL-2 therapy,

intravesically delivered IFN-α has been established as well-tolerated by patients and is likely well-tolerated even through gene therapy.

Preclinical studies conducted by Iqbal Ahmed and colleagues[38] in 2001 found that recombinant adenovirus expressing human IFN-α2b could generate biologically active IFN expression in both rat models as well as in vitro. Recombinant Ad-IFN-α2b was also able to generate an antitumor response in xenografts. Benedict and colleagues[39] subsequently demonstrated that intravesical instillation of adenovirus-encoding IFN-α along with Syn3 into athymic mouse models growing KY7/GFP human bladder tumors led to marked tumor regression. High levels of IFN protein were identified in both urine and bladder tissue after intravesical exposure. Cytotoxicity to bladder cancer cell lines were demonstrated after Ad-IFN instillation, and IFN levels were noted for at least 7 days after treatment. This data provided some of the initial steps justifying further evaluation of using intravesical Ad-IFN-α/Syn3 to treat NMIBC (see **Fig. 1**).[39]

Several questions remained. First, how did IFN-based gene therapy generate tumor cell cytotoxicity? Izawa and colleagues[40] answered this question in part with data that demonstrated that IFN triggered an indirect antiangiogenic effect, caused in part by downregulating the expression

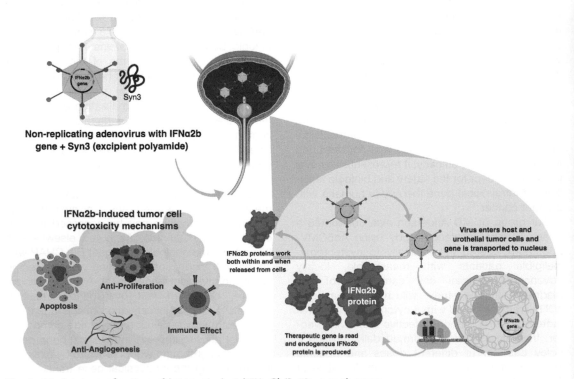

Fig. 1. Mechanisms of action of intravesical rAdIFN-α2b/Syn3 gene therapy.

of the angiogenesis factors basic fibroblast growth factor and matrix metalloproteinase-9 within tumor cells. Neovascularization of tumor cells was therefore restricted, and secondarily led to tumor cell apoptosis. A second component of IFN-stimulated cytotoxicity is driven by TRAIL-mediated apoptosis, which Papageorgiou and colleagues[41] reported occurred through an IRF-1–dependent mechanism. Indeed, elevated TRAIL levels have also been noted in patients with detectable urinary IFN-α levels after treatment.[42] A second question related to selection of the appropriate dosing strategy when using Ad-IFN-α intravesically. Tao and colleagues[43] showed that single instillations were just as effective as sequential instillations and identified a dosing floor using an orthotopic bladder cancer model. A dose of 1×10^{11} particles/mL along with Syn3 was found to be effective in decreasing the size of tumors.[44]

HUMAN TRIALS USING ADENOVIRUS-MEDIATED INTERFERON-BASED GENE THERAPY

The results of the first phase I clinical trial evaluating the safety and toxicity of intravesical rAd-IFN-α/Syn3 was published in 2013.[45] In the study, patients with non–muscle-invasive disease (Ta, Tis, T1) who had recurred following at least 2 cycles of BCG were enrolled to receive 1 of 5 dosing cohorts, using a standard dose-escalation design. Patients were monitored daily for adverse events up to 5 days after treatment, and after 12 weeks of therapy, underwent cystoscopy with bladder biopsy and urine cytology. A total of 17 patients were enrolled in the study. No dose-limiting toxicities were identified, nor were there any significant treatment-related adverse events. The most common complaints after therapy included urinary urgency, headache, fatigue, and nausea. Lower urinary tract symptoms, which were encountered by 88% of patients, were well-managed with anticholinergic therapy. The efficiency of gene therapy was assessed by detecting levels of IFN-α protein in the urine. All but the lowest dose were able to generate detectable IFN-α protein levels. Out of the 14 patients treated with effective dosing and who had confirmed gene transfer (as evidenced by detectable urinary IFN-α), 6 (43%) had a CR at 3 months, with 2 remaining disease free at 29 and 39 months.

In the phase II setting, conducted between 2012 and 2015 by the Society of Urologic Oncology Clinical Trials Consortium, 40 patients from 13 centers with a diagnosis of high-grade BCG-refractory or relapsed NMIBC (Ta, Tis, T1) were randomized to receive either a low dose (1×10^{11} viral particles/mL) or high dose (3×10^{11} viral particles/mL) of rAdIFN-α/Syn3 intravesically.[46] The study was multi-institutional and patients were treated every 3 months for 1 year, at which point they received a study-mandated biopsy from the location of the index tumor and at least 5 random bladder biopsies from protocol-specified locations. The primary end point of the phase II trial was 25% freedom from high-grade recurrence at 12 months, and evidence of effective gene transfer was found in all trial patients as determined by measurable levels of IFN-α-2b in the urine of patients. There seemed to be no significant difference between the 2 dosing arms, although the median time to recurrence slightly favored the high-dose group (6.5 mo vs 3.5 mo). Importantly, rAdIFN-α/Syn3 seemed to act on both papillary and CIS BCG-unresponsive lesions; a subset analysis demonstrated a 50% high-grade recurrence-free survival rate for papillary tumors at 12 months, and a 30% high-grade recurrence-free survival rate for CIS lesions. The latter is particularly important given the paucity of treatment options available for patients with CIS; the only approved agent aside from BCG remains valrubicin, which has only a 10% RFS rate at 12 months.[47] Long-term follow-up data from the phase II trial are pending.

In late 2016, a multi-institutional phase III trial for rAdIFN-α/Syn3 (Adstiladrin, previously Instiladrin) was initiated to evaluate the efficacy of the therapy in treating patients with high-grade BCG-unresponsive non–muscle-invasive disease, 100 of whom must have CIS. In addition to determining the CR rate as well as CR-durability among patients with CIS, the trial seeks to understand the percent of high-grade recurrence-free survival at 3-month intervals up to 1 year in patients with Ta/T1 lesions without CIS. This trial completed accrual in the second quarter of 2018 and data are maturing.

ONGOING EFFORTS TO OPTIMIZE INTERFERON-BASED GENE THERAPY

The role of combination therapy with gene therapy constructs is currently unknown and an area of ongoing area interest to our group. Plote and colleagues[48] evaluated the immunologic mechanisms that mediated IFN-stimulated immune responses using poly:IC, a toll-like receptor 3 agonist that acts as a synthetic analogue of IFN. Among the key findings included the fact that IFN drives an inflammatory response driven by both innate and adaptive immune cells, including increased CD8 T cells, natural killer cells, and CD11b⁺Ly6G⁺ cells.[48] In addition, mice containing MB49 urothelial tumors that were treated with a combination of poly:IC and anti–PD-1 monoclonal antibody showed prolonged survival, decreased angiogenesis, and enhanced MAPK/AKT signaling.[48] Thus, efforts to combine immune checkpoint inhibitors along with intravesical viral-mediated IFN may further potentiate an antitumor response and warrant additional study.

Our laboratory is also investigating the role of urine-derived biomarkers after treatment with intravesical gene therapy to better predict which patients may most benefit from intravesical gene therapy. An analysis of the immune cells that are shed within the urine of patients with NMIBC may provide an opportunity to identify patients who would most benefit from a cytokine-based intravesical treatment versus an alternative form of therapy. Correlative data from the phase I and II rAdIFN-α/Syn3 studies are being used to explore the role of urinary biomarkers further.

Finally, the use of vectors other than adenovirus are also under investigation. Lentivirus in particular holds promise. Lentivirus is more efficient than adenovirus at viral transfection, in part owing to its ability to infect nondividing cells. Further, lentiviral IFN constructs can integrate into the host's genome to allow for the continual production and sustained release of IFN-α. Preliminary data, recently presented at the 2019 Genitourinary Cancers symposium, showed that LV-IFN-α effectively increases the expression of IFN-α in vitro and in vivo along with concomitant TRAIL-mediated cytotoxicity to infected urothelial cancer cells. Efforts at further elucidating the mechanism of this agent remain ongoing.[49]

OTHER INTRAVESICAL GENE THERAPY AGENTS UNDER INVESTIGATION

CG0070 is a replication-competent adenovirus that selectively replicates in Rb pathway-defective bladder tumor cells, in addition to stimulating the expression of granulocyte-macrophage colony-stimulating factor. Burke and colleagues[50] reported the results of a phase I study in which CG0070 was administered to 35 patients with recurrent NMIBC after at least 1 prior course of intravesical BCG. Patients received either a single dose or multidose intravesical course, and safety was assessed. The agent was found to have no dose-limiting toxicities with the most frequently reported adverse event being dysuria. CR was achieved in only 50% of patients with CIS (4 of 8 patients), and in 41.2% of patients with CIS with or without Ta/T1 (7 of 17 patients).[50] All patients had high detectable levels of granulocyte-macrophage colony-stimulating factor in the urine after treatment.[50]

In the phase II setting, CG0070 was administered 14 days after the most recent biopsy in patients with NMIBC (Ta, T1, CIS) who were BCG-unresponsive and had refused cystectomy.[51] The agent was coinstilled with 0.1% dodecyl maltoside, a nonionic surfactant used to enhance transduction (similar to the role played by Syn3 in the rAdIFN studies). Therapy was administered intravesically every week for 6 weeks for both induction and maintenance courses. At 3 months, 2 patients had progressed to muscle-invasive disease, 1 patient had baseline persistence of CIS, and the other had T1 disease.[51] At 6 months, the CR rate was 47%, which included a 58% CR rate for pure CIS.[51] The 12-month data have yet to be published, but interim results

Table 1
Key clinical studies involving intravesical gene therapy

Author, Year	Setting	Agent	Patient Population
Kuball et al,[32] 2002	Phase I	rAd-p53 (SCH-58500)	MIBC patients scheduled for RC
Pagliaro et al,[34] 2003	Phase I	rAd5-CMV-p53	Cystectomy-ineligible locally advanced UCC
Burke et al,[50] 2012	Phase I	CG0070	Recurrent NMIBC after ≥1 prior intravesical BCG dose
Dinney et al,[45] 2013	Phase I	rAdIFN-α2b/Syn3	BCG-unresponsive patients with NMIBC
Shore et al,[46] 2017	Phase II	rAdIFN-α2b/Syn3	BCG-unresponsive patients with NMIBC
Packiam et al,[51] 2018	Phase II	CG0070	BCG-unresponsive patients with NMIBC who had refused cystectomy

Abbreviations: CMV, cytomegalovirus; MIBC, muscle-invasive bladder cancer; RC, radical cystectomy; UCC, urothelial cell carcinoma.

were reported at the 2018 American Urologic Association Annual Meeting; the CR rate was noted to be 30%, with CIS-containing tumors having a 27% CR (n = 45), whereas pure Ta/T1 tumors had a 38% CR (n = 16). Ten patients underwent cystectomy, of whom 6 patients were found to have progressed to muscle-invasive disease.[52] **Table 1** summarizes the key clinical studies published to date investigating the use of intravesical gene therapy for bladder cancer.

SUMMARY

BCG-unresponsive NMIBC remains a challenging disease to treat. Intravesical gene therapy represents a promising novel approach to management and will likely expand to include combination therapies. Additional insights into the mechanisms that underlie intravesical gene transduction and immune modulation, along with a more granular understanding of the molecular defects that occur in NMIBC tumor biology are also likely to provide us with additional therapeutic targets in the future.

REFERENCES

1. van den Bosch S, Alfred Witjes J. Long-term cancer-specific survival in patients with high-risk, non-muscle-invasive bladder cancer and tumour progression: a systematic review. Eur Urol 2011;60(3): 493–500.
2. Chamie K, Litwin MS, Bassett JC, et al. Recurrence of high-risk bladder cancer: a population-based analysis. Cancer 2013;119(17):3219–27.
3. Pearl R. Cancer and tuberculosis. Am J Hyg 1929;9: 97–159.
4. Morales A, Eidinger D, Bruce AW. Intracavitary Bacillus Calmette-Guerin in the treatment of superficial bladder tumors. J Urol 1976;116(2):180–3. Available at: http://www.ncbi.nlm.nih.gov/pubmed/820877.
5. Ratliff TL, Kavoussi LR, Catalona WJ. Role of fibronectin in intravesical BCG therapy for superficial bladder cancer. J Urol 1988;139(2):410–4. Available at: http://www.ncbi.nlm.nih.gov/pubmed/3276931.
6. Jackson AM, Alexandroff AB, Kelly RW, et al. Changes in urinary cytokines and soluble intercellular adhesion molecule-1 (ICAM-1) in bladder cancer patients after bacillus Calmette-Guérin (BCG) immunotherapy. Clin Exp Immunol 1995;99(3): 369–75. Available at: http://www.ncbi.nlm.nih.gov/pubmed/7882559.
7. Fuge O, Vasdev N, Allchorne P, et al. Immunotherapy for bladder cancer. Res Rep Urol 2015;7: 65–79.
8. Buffen K, Oosting M, Quintin J, et al. Autophagy controls BCG-induced trained immunity and the response to intravesical BCG therapy for bladder cancer. PLoS Pathog 2014;10(10):e1004485.
9. Morales A, Ottenhof P, Emerson L. Treatment of residual, non-infiltrating bladder cancer with bacillus Calmette-Guerin. J Urol 1981;125(5): 649–51. Available at: http://www.ncbi.nlm.nih.gov/pubmed/7014931.
10. Lamm DL, Blumenstein BA, Crissman JD, et al. Maintenance bacillus Calmette-Guerin immunotherapy for recurrent TA, T1 and carcinoma in situ transitional cell carcinoma of the bladder: a randomized Southwest Oncology Group Study. J Urol 2000; 163(4):1124–9. Available at: http://www.ncbi.nlm.nih.gov/pubmed/10737480.
11. Lamm DL. Long-term results of intravesical therapy for superficial bladder cancer. Urol Clin North Am 1992;19(3):573–80. Available at: http://www.ncbi.nlm.nih.gov/pubmed/1636241.
12. Choi W, Porten S, Kim S, et al. Identification of Distinct Basal and Luminal Subtypes of Muscle-Invasive Bladder Cancer with Different Sensitivities to Frontline Chemotherapy. Cancer Cell 2014;25(2): 152–65.
13. Damrauer JS, Hoadley KA, Chism DD, et al. Intrinsic subtypes of high-grade bladder cancer reflect the hallmarks of breast cancer biology. Proc Natl Acad Sci U S A 2014;111(8):3110–5.
14. Cancer Genome Atlas Research Network. Comprehensive molecular characterization of urothelial bladder carcinoma. Nature 2014;507(7492):315–22.
15. Allory Y, Beukers W, Sagrera A, et al. Telomerase reverse transcriptase promoter mutations in bladder cancer: high frequency across stages, detection in urine, and lack of association with outcome. Eur Urol 2014;65(2):360–6.
16. Cappellen D, De Oliveira C, Ricol D, et al. Frequent activating mutations of FGFR3 in human bladder and cervix carcinomas. Nat Genet 1999;23(1): 18–20.
17. Zieger K, Dyrskjøt L, Wiuf C, et al. Role of activating fibroblast growth factor receptor 3 mutations in the development of bladder tumors. Clin Cancer Res 2005;11(21):7709–19.
18. Hernández S, López-Knowles E, Lloreta J, et al. Prospective study of FGFR3 mutations as a prognostic factor in nonmuscle invasive urothelial bladder carcinomas. J Clin Oncol 2006;24(22):3664–71.
19. Platt FM, Hurst CD, Taylor CF, et al. Spectrum of phosphatidylinositol 3-kinase pathway gene alterations in bladder cancer. Clin Cancer Res 2009; 15(19):6008–17.
20. Taylor CF, Platt FM, Hurst CD, et al. Frequent inactivating mutations of STAG2 in bladder cancer are associated with low tumour grade and stage and inversely related to chromosomal copy number changes. Hum Mol Genet 2014;23(8): 1964–74.

21. Hurst CD, Alder O, Platt FM, et al. Genomic Subtypes of Non-invasive Bladder Cancer with Distinct Metabolic Profile and Female Gender Bias in KDM6A Mutation Frequency. Cancer Cell 2017; 32(5):701–15.e7.

22. Mulligan RC. The basic science of gene therapy. Science 1993;260(5110):926–32. Available at: http://www.ncbi.nlm.nih.gov/pubmed/8493530.

23. Wirth T, Parker N, Ylä-Herttuala S. History of gene therapy. Gene 2013;525(2):162–9.

24. Duplisea JJ, Mokkapati S, Plote D, et al. The development of interferon-based gene therapy for BCG unresponsive bladder cancer: from bench to bedside. World J Urol 2018. https://doi.org/10.1007/s00345-018-2553-7.

25. Kaji EH, Leiden JM. Gene and stem cell therapies. JAMA 2001;285(5):545–50. Available at: http://www.ncbi.nlm.nih.gov/pubmed/11176856.

26. Esrig D, Elmajian D, Groshen S, et al. Accumulation of nuclear p53 and tumor progression in bladder cancer. N Engl J Med 1994;331(19):1259–64.

27. Takahashi R, Hashimoto T, Xu HJ, et al. The retinoblastoma gene functions as a growth and tumor suppressor in human bladder carcinoma cells. Proc Natl Acad Sci U S A 1991;88(12):5257–61. Available at: http://www.ncbi.nlm.nih.gov/pubmed/2052605.

28. Pagliaro LC, Keyhani A, Liu B, et al. Adenoviral p53 gene transfer in human bladder cancer cell lines: cytotoxicity and synergy with cisplatin. Urol Oncol 2003;21(6):456–62. Available at: http://www.ncbi.nlm.nih.gov/pubmed/14693272.

29. Pagliaro LC. Gene therapy for bladder cancer. World J Urol 2000;18(2):148–51. Available at: http://www.ncbi.nlm.nih.gov/pubmed/10854151.

30. Zhang WW, Fang X, Mazur W, et al. High-efficiency gene transfer and high-level expression of wild-type p53 in human lung cancer cells mediated by recombinant adenovirus. Cancer Gene Ther 1994;1(1):5–13. Available at: http://www.ncbi.nlm.nih.gov/pubmed/7621238.

31. Morris BD, Drazan KE, Csete ME, et al. Adenoviral-mediated gene transfer to bladder in vivo. J Urol 1994;152(2 Pt 1):506–9. Available at: http://www.ncbi.nlm.nih.gov/pubmed/8015103.

32. Kuball J, Wen SF, Leissner J, et al. Successful adenovirus-mediated wild-type p53 gene transfer in patients with bladder cancer by intravesical vector instillation. J Clin Oncol 2002;20(4):957–65.

33. Connor RJ, Engler H, Machemer T, et al. Identification of polyamides that enhance adenovirus-mediated gene expression in the urothelium. Gene Ther 2001;8(1):41–8.

34. Pagliaro LC, Keyhani A, Williams D, et al. Repeated intravesical instillations of an adenoviral vector in patients with locally advanced bladder cancer: a phase I study of p53 gene therapy. J Clin Oncol 2003;21(12):2247–53.

35. Klingler CH. Glycosaminoglycans: how much do we know about their role in the bladder? Urologia 2016; 83(Suppl 1):11–4.

36. Yamashita M, Rosser CJ, Zhou J-H, et al. Syn3 provides high levels of intravesical adenoviral-mediated gene transfer for gene therapy of genetically altered urothelium and superficial bladder cancer. Cancer Gene Ther 2002;9(8):687–91.

37. Joudi FN, Smith BJ, O'Donnell MA, National BCG-Interferon Phase 2 Investigator Group. Final results from a national multicenter phase II trial of combination bacillus Calmette-Guérin plus interferon alpha-2B for reducing recurrence of superficial bladder cancer. Urol Oncol 2006;24(4):344–8.

38. Iqbal Ahmed CM, Johnson DE, Demers GW, et al. Interferon alpha2b gene delivery using adenoviral vector causes inhibition of tumor growth in xenograft models from a variety of cancers. Cancer Gene Ther 2001;8(10):788–95.

39. Benedict WF, Tao Z, Kim C-S, et al. Intravesical Ad-IFNalpha causes marked regression of human bladder cancer growing orthotopically in nude mice and overcomes resistance to IFN-alpha protein. Mol Ther 2004;10(3):525–32.

40. Izawa JI, Sweeney P, Perrotte P, et al. Inhibition of tumorigenicity and metastasis of human bladder cancer growing in athymic mice by interferon-beta gene therapy results partially from various antiangiogenic effects including endothelial cell apoptosis. Clin Cancer Res 2002;8(4):1258–70. Available at: http://www.ncbi.nlm.nih.gov/pubmed/11948141.

41. Papageorgiou A, Dinney CPN, McConkey DJ. Interferon-alpha induces TRAIL expression and cell death via an IRF-1-dependent mechanism in human bladder cancer cells. Cancer Biol Ther 2007;6(6):872–9. Available at: http://www.ncbi.nlm.nih.gov/pubmed/17617740.

42. Benedict WF, Fisher M, Zhang X-Q, et al. Use of monitoring levels of soluble forms of cytokeratin 18 in the urine of patients with superficial bladder cancer following intravesical Ad-IFNα/Syn3 treatment in a phase I study. Cancer Gene Ther 2014;21(3):91–4.

43. Tao Z, Connor RJ, Ashoori F, et al. Efficacy of a single intravesical treatment with Ad-IFN/Syn 3 is dependent on dose and urine IFN concentration obtained: implications for clinical investigation. Cancer Gene Ther 2006;13(2):125–30.

44. Connor RJ, Anderson JM, Machemer T, et al. Sustained intravesical interferon protein exposure is achieved using an adenoviral-mediated gene delivery system: a study in rats evaluating dosing regimens. Urology 2005;66(1):224–9.

45. Dinney CPN, Fisher MB, Navai N, et al. Phase I trial of intravesical recombinant adenovirus mediated interferon-α2b formulated in Syn3 for Bacillus Calmette-Guérin failures in nonmuscle invasive bladder cancer. J Urol 2013;190(3):850–6.

46. Shore ND, Boorjian SA, Canter DJ, et al. Intravesical rAd-IFNα/Syn3 for patients with high-grade, bacillus Calmette-Guerin-refractory or relapsed non-muscle-invasive bladder cancer: a phase II randomized study. J Clin Oncol 2017;35(30):3410–6.

47. Dinney CPN, Greenberg RE, Steinberg GD. Intravesical valrubicin in patients with bladder carcinoma in situ and contraindication to or failure after bacillus Calmette-Guérin. Urol Oncol 2013;31(8):1635–42.

48. Plote D, Choi W, Mokkapati S, et al. Inhibition of urothelial carcinoma through targeted type I interferon-mediated immune activation. Oncoimmunology 2019;8(5):e1577125.

49. Mokkapati S, Duplisea JJ, Plote D, et al. Lentiviral interferon: a novel method for gene therapy in bladder cancer. J Clin Oncol 2019;(Suppl 7S) [abstract: 456].

50. Burke JM, Lamm DL, Meng MV, et al. A first in human phase 1 study of CG0070, a GM-CSF expressing oncolytic adenovirus, for the treatment of nonmuscle invasive bladder cancer. J Urol 2012;188(6):2391–7.

51. Packiam VT, Lamm DL, Barocas DA, et al. An open label, single-arm, phase II multicenter study of the safety and efficacy of CG0070 oncolytic vector regimen in patients with BCG-unresponsive non-muscle-invasive bladder cancer: interim results. Urol Oncol 2018;36(10):440–7.

52. Packiam VT, Barocas DA, Chamie K, et al. LBA24 CG0070, an oncolytic adenovirus, for bcg-unresponsive non-muscle-invasive bladder cancer (NMIBC): 12 month interim results from a multicenter phase II trial. J Urol 2018;199(4S). https://doi.org/10.1016/j.juro.2018.03.096.

Immuno-Oncology Approaches to Salvage Treatment for Non-muscle invasive Bladder Cancer

Niranjan J. Sathianathen, MD[a,b,c,*], Subodh Regmi, MD[a],
Shilpa Gupta, MD[d], Badrinath R. Konety, MD, MBA[a]

KEYWORDS

- Bladder cancer • Immunotherapy • Oncology • Non–muscle-invasive bladder cancer

KEY POINTS

- There is a complex interplay between bladder cancer and immune cells such as myeloid-derived suppressor cells, neutrophils, tumor-associated macrophages, and T lymphocytes that can be harnessed as targets for therapy.
- Early results show promise for checkpoint inhibitors, recombinant interferon-α2b protein and oncolytic adenoviruses to be used as a salvage treatment after bacillus Calmette-Guérin in non–muscle-invasive disease.
- The currently available data are in early stages and maturation is awaited to improve understanding of the optimal immunotherapy agent to be used as salvage treatment in non–muscle-Invasive disease.

Approximately three-quarters of all newly diagnosed bladder cancers are nonmuscle invasive. The gold standard management option for non–muscle-invasive bladder cancer (NMIBC) is transurethral resection followed by intravesical chemotherapy or immunotherapy to decrease the risk of recurrence.[1] Chemotherapeutic agents, such as mitomycin C and gemcitabine, are used for low-risk NMIBC; whereas bacillus Calmette-Guérin (BCG) immunotherapy is used for intermediate- and high-risk disease. Although these agents have been demonstrated to decrease the risk of recurrence in large phase III randomized trials, a large proportion of patients still experience recurrent disease. The management of chemorefractory and BCG-refractory disease is an important area of research in the NMIBC domain. As with other malignancies refractory or unresponsive to traditional therapies, systemic therapy with a new generation of immuno-oncology agents have or are being investigated for used as salvage therapy in this setting. We provide a comprehensive review of the current evidence in this area and provide a window into what lies ahead in the future.

Disclosure Statement: The authors have nothing to disclose.
[a] Department of Urology, University of Minnesota, 420 Delaware Street Southeast, MMC 394, Minneapolis, MN, USA; [b] Department of Surgery, The University of Melbourne, Parkville, Victoria, Australia; [c] Department of Cancer Surgery, Peter MacCallum Cancer Centre, Parkville, Victoria, Australia; [d] Department of Hematology and Oncology, Taussig Cancer Institute, Cleveland Clinic Foundation, Cleveland, Ohio, USA
* Corresponding author.
E-mail address: nsathian@umn.edu
Twitter: @NiranjanJS (N.J.S.)

Urol Clin N Am 47 (2020) 103–110
https://doi.org/10.1016/j.ucl.2019.09.012

BLADDER CANCER AND THE IMMUNE SYSTEM

The relationship between cancer processes and the immune system is incredibly complex and cannot be fully explored in this limited space, but we aim to provide a overview of this interplay.

Bladder cancer often causes local inflammation and consequently attracts inflammatory cells to the site. However, the local immunosuppression caused by neoplastic processes results in these cells being unable to combat the cancer. Myeloid-derived suppressor cell are a cell type that has been implicated in cancer-associated immunosuppression. Several preclinical studies have demonstrated that the increased concentration of myeloid-derived suppressor cells in peripheral blood and tumor tissue potentiates cancer progression through immune suppression and stimulation of angiogenesis.[2] Eruslanov and colleagues[3] found an increased number of granulocyte-type $CD15^{high}CD33^{low}$ cells in peripheral blood and tumor tissue in patients with bladder cancer compared with healthy controls. Monocyte-type $CD15^{low}CD33^{high}$ cells were also found in these patients but their concentration was not markedly higher than in controls. However, both the aforementioned cell types were highly activated and produced considerable amounts of proinflammatory chemokines and cytokines. These findings can be potential targets of immunotherapies to induce quiescence of the overactivated states of myeloid-derived suppressor cells and their immunosuppressive effects.

Neutrophils have also been implicated in promoting bladder cancer growth. Human neutrophil proteins (HNP)-1, -2, and -3 have been shown to promote tumor cell growth through the recruitment of leukocytes across a range of malignancies.[4] They may have additional roles, such as the inhibition of angiogenesis and immunomodulation, which may all contribute to tumor invasion. Higher levels of HNPs have been found in the urine and serum of patients with bladder cancer compared with controls.[5,6] Furthermore, Gunes and colleagues[5] demonstrated that plasma levels of HNPs were greater in patients with more aggressive cancers such as patients with metastatic disease and nodal involvement. The method in which HNPs exert their tumorigenic effects are not completely clear and need further research to be understood.

The role of tumor-associated macrophages (TAMs) in cancer development and progress has been extensively studied.[7] Several studies have reported that the presence of TAMs in malignant tissue is associated with a poorer prognosis.[8] The role of TAMs in potentiating tumor growth is all encompassing and has been reported to involve inhibiting the T-cell–mediated immune response and stimulating angiogenesis, cell proliferation, and metastasis. As can be seen with their many functions, TAMs are complex cells and are involved with various immune pathways. To simplify it, we can consider TAMS as having 2 phenotypical forms: M1 and M2. M1 phenotype has antitumor effects by slowing cell proliferation and causes tissue damage. In contrast, the M2 phenotype promotes tumor growth by causing immunosuppression, angiogenesis, and promoting invasion. Lima and colleagues[9] demonstrated that patients who experienced BCG failure had higher concentration of M2 TAMs in their stroma relative to tumor tissue compared with those who had a successful response to BCG. This pattern of TAMs was associated with poorer prognosis as patients with higher M2 TAMs in their stroma had decreased recurrence-free survival. Ajili and colleagues[10] also found that TAMs were associated with BCG failure. These findings have been validated in further studies, which found that $CD163^+$ TAM infiltration was associated with increased vascular invasion and distant metastasis.[11] Although Xu and colleagues[11] did not find that TAMs were directly associated with worse overall survival and recurrence-free survival, they did find a positive correlation between $CD163^+$ TAM infiltration and B7-H3 expression; the latter conferred worse survival. Hanada and colleagues[12] reported that higher TAM counts are associated with muscle-invasive disease and higher rates of radical cystectomy in addition to worse 5-year survival.

T lymphocytes have an important role in tumor development and progression. Regulatory T cells have been shown to be involved in modulating the immune response in maintaining self-tolerance. They have the ability to downregulate the antitumor immune response and therefore potential cancer growth and spread.[13] High concentrations of regulatory T cells in tumor tissue is associated with a worse prognosis. BCG exerts a part of its action against bladder cancer through the regulation of T cells and natural killer cells. Furthermore, IL-2, which is produced by T lymphocytes, has been shown to be associated with higher recurrence of bladder cancer. Although the evidence in bladder cancer is somewhat limited, it is evident that T lymphocytes are intrinsically linked to tumorigenesis in the bladder. Therefore, T lymphocytes could be a target of immunotherapy.

EMERGING IMMUNOTHERAPIES FOR SALVAGE TREATMENT OF NON–MUSCLE-INVASIVE BLADDER CANCER

The use of immuno-oncology in BCG-unresponsive disease is a developing area and the evidence is in its infancy. In an attempt to avoid, or at least, delay surgical removal of the bladder, a number of trials have evaluated using a variety of agents for BCG refractory disease. The majority of trials have shown very little success and, as a result, we continue the search for other therapies to use in this setting. Several of the studies discussed elsewhere in this article did not administer patients with adequate BCG (as defined by the US Food and Drug Administration consensus recommendations) initially which entails at least 5 of 6 weekly instillations of induction therapy, 2 of 3 instillations of maintenance therapy or a re-induction course of at least 5 of 6 instillations. Therefore, we are extrapolating the effect of the below mentioned agents after inadequate BCG to the true BCG refractory setting.

Although there are several ongoing trials, only a limited number have reported their results, which are discussed here.

Checkpoint inhibitors have been a revelation in the field of immunotherapy across several tumors. As mentioned elsewhere in this article, T cells have a role in attenuating the immune response to malignant cells. Checkpoint

inhibitors work by counteracting this and reestablishing the ability of the immune system to attack cancer cells (**Fig. 1**). Programmed death ligand-1 (PD-L1), programmed cell death protein-1, and cytotoxic T-lymphocyte associated protein 4 are 3 of the main targets of checkpoint inhibitors in bladder cancer. Early preclinical studies demonstrated that the binding of PD-L1 to programmed cell death protein-1 on activated T and B cells resulted in immunosuppression. Therefore, it is suggested that inhibition of this ligand and/or protein should reactivate the immune system. Pembrolizumab is an anti–programmed cell death protein-1 antibody that was first shown to have benefit in advanced cancers including melanoma, non-small cell lung cancer, and even urothelial carcinoma. Specifically to NMIBC, BCG interacts with these pathways. Chevalier and colleagues[14] found that the administration of BCG resulted in increased levels of PD-L1+ regulatory T cells urine and could possibly be an important mechanism in BCG-refractory disease. These findings are supported by a study by Hashizume and colleagues[15] in which tissue microarrays before and after BCG instillation were stained by antibodies against PD-L1, PD-L2, and CD8; and showed that PD-L1 expression was significantly increased on tumor cell, tumor-infiltrating inflammatory cells, and inflammatory cells after BCG therapy. A single-arm phase II trial (KEYNOTE-057, NCT02625961) administered pembrolizumab to 101 patients with histologically confirmed

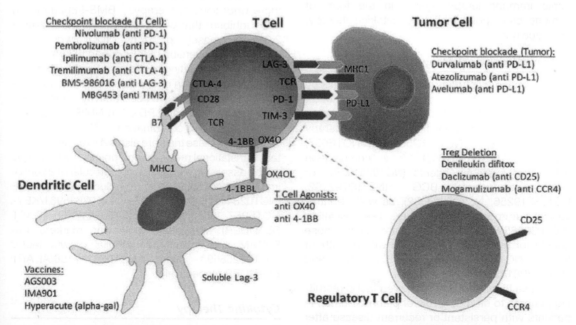

Fig. 1. Action of immunotherapy agents on immune cells. (*From* Ball MW, Allaf ME, Drake CG. Recent advances in immunotherapy for kidney cancer. Discovery medicine. 2016;21:305-13; with permission.)

high-grade BCG-unresponsive NMIBC and found that the complete response rate at 3 months was 41.2%.[16–18] Of those patients who experienced a complete response, the mean duration of response was 8.1 months, 85.6% had a response for longer than 6 months, and 57% had a response beyond 12 months.[18] Furthermore, the majority of complete responders had an ongoing response at a median of 21 months of follow-up. No patients experienced progression to muscle-invasive disease. It should be noted that 15.5% of the cohort experienced an immune-mediated side effect, including 2.1% who experienced grade III or IV toxicities. The results of this trial provide encouragement for the use of checkpoint inhibitors in BCG-refractory disease, which are being evaluated in several other studies, which are discussed elsewhere in this article.

ONGOING TRIALS AND FUTURE DIRECTIONS

There are several ongoing trials that are investigating the role of salvage therapies in patients who have failed to respond to intravesical BCG. Immunotherapy as a treatment category has important presence in the salvage setting as well as in patients who are BCG naïve. Systemic immunotherapy in the form of immune check point inhibitors look most promising with several trials showing benefits in the locally advanced as well as metastatic setting.[19,20]

Three forms of immunotherapy are being evaluated in current clinical trials. These include systemic immunotherapy agents in the form of immune checkpoint inhibitors, cytokine therapy, and vaccines.

Systemic Immunotherapy Agents

Several phase I/II studies are studying the efficacy of pembrolizumab, atezolizumab, duravulumab, and nivolumab (**Table 1**). These agents are being studied as a standalone systemic therapy (NCT02324582, NCT02625961/KEYNOTE057, NCT02844816/SWOG1605),[21,22] in combination with other systemic agents (NCT03519256) or with intravesical BCG (NCT02792192, NCT03519256, NCT02324582), as well as intravesical immunologic agents like vicinium (NCT03258593). Some trials are using these agents for intravesical instillation with or without BCG (NCT02808143, NCT03759496, and NCT02808143).

A phase III randomized controlled trial is recruiting patients to study the role of pembrolizumab in patients with persistent or recurrent disease after adequate BCG induction. This study is designed to assess the antitumor efficacy and safety of pembrolizumab in combination with BCG in comparison with BCG monotherapy with the primary hypothesis that the combination of pembrolizumab plus BCG has a superior complete response rate compared with BCG in participants with carcinoma in situ (NCT03711032/KEYNOTE676).

KEYNOTE057 (NCT02625961) and SWOG1605 (NCT28448216) share similar trial designs and end points, but are using pembrolizumab and atezolizumab, respectively. Similarly, NCT02324582, which is a phase I study looking at the safety and efficacy of administering a 200 mg fixed dose of pembrolizumab in conjunction with intravesical BCG treatment, is nearing completion. NCT02808143 is a phase I dose escalation study of intravesical pembrolizumab and bacillus Calmette-Guerin (BCG), which is expected to complete by early 2020. The ADAPT BLADDER trial (NCT03317158) is a 2-phased study where the aim is to determine the optimal dosing for durvalumab in combination with BCG and external beam radiotherapy in phase I. In phase II, the aim is to compare the outcomes between Durvalumab + BCG, Durvalumab + external beam radiotherapy and retreatment with BCG only in patients who have relapsed with prior BCG therapy. CheckMate 9UT (NCT03519256) is a phase II, randomized, open-label study assessing the safety and efficacy of nivolumab with or without BMS-986205 with or without intravesical BCG.[23] The rationale is based on the results seen with immunotherapy-naive advanced patients with bladder cancer who had received 1 or more prior lines of therapy.[24] BMS-986205 is an IDO1 inhibitor that works in the IDO (indoleamine 2,3-dioxygenase) pathway. IDO works by enhancing conversion of tryptophan to kynurenine and thereby depleting tryptophan levels, which results in suppression of effector T cells and promotion of regulatory T-cell activity. Increased expression of IDO and PD-L1 in NMIBC supports the testing of this combination.[25,26]

Several of these trials are also set to assess important translational medicine end points,[27] where they will be assessing expression of molecular markers of immune checkpoint blockade including PD-L1, CD8 (NCT02844816/SWOG1605, NCT02625961/KEYNOTE057, NCT03258593, NCT033117158/ADAPT BLADDER) and other molecular markers like EpCAM and vascular endothelial growth factor (NCT03258593 and NCT033117158/ADAPT BLADDER respectively).

Cytokine Therapy

The beneficial effects of IL-2 therapy in the treatment of melanoma[28] formed the basis for most

Table 1
List of current immuno-oncology trials with PD-1 inhibitors in salvage setting for NMIBC

Drug/Route	Trial ID	Phase	Estimated/ Enrolled Number	Outcomes	Completion Date
Pembrolizumab IV	NCT02324582	I (single arm)	15	Primary: Safety/ efficacy Secondary: CRR, change in QOL	January 2021
Pembrolizumab intravesical with BCG	NCT02808143	I (single arm)	27	Primary: maximal tolerated dose Secondary: Incidence of adverse events, dose limiting toxicity Others: Pharmacokinetics, humoral and cellular responses	February 2021
Pembrolizumab IV	NCT02625961 KEYNOTE057	II (single arm)	260	Primary: CRR, DFS (up to 3 y) Secondary: duration of response	July 2023
Pembrolizumab with Intravesical BCG vs Intravesical BCG only	NCT03711032 KEYNOTE676	III (RCT)	550	Primary: CRR (up to 3.5 y) In CIS Secondary: EFS, RFS, OS, DSS, time to cystectomy, QoL	November 2024
Atezolizumab IV ± BCG	NCT02792192	Ib/IIa (nonrando-mized)	24	Primary: percentage with adverse events, CR Secondary: duration of CR, % RFS, PFS, CFS, OS	November 2021
Atezolizumab IV	NCT02844816 SWOG 1605	II (single arm)	162	Primary: CR at 25 wk, EFS Secondary: PFS, EFS in Ta/T1, CFS, BCSS Tertiary: CR in CIS, PDL-1 and CD8 expression, immune signature expression.	February 2020
Durvalumab IV + Vicinium Intravesical	NCT03258593	I	40	Primary: safety and tolerability Secondary: Biomarkers of immune response, pharmacokinetics, urine EpCAM, PDL-1 expression, PD-1 expressing T Cells	July 2021

(continued on next page)

Table 1
(continued)

Drug/Route	Trial ID	Phase	Estimated/ Enrolled Number	Outcomes	Completion Date
Durvalumab IV vs combos with BCG and EBRT	NCT03317158 ADAPT BLADDER	I → II (Randomized with crossover)	186	Phase I—Primary: determine the dose of combos Secondary: RLFR sat 6 mo, safety of mono/doublet treatments Phase II—Primary: RFLS at 6 mo Secondary: 24 mo RLFS, PD-1 expression and association with RLFS, safety profile	September 2021
Durvalumab Intravesical	NCT03759496	II	39	Primary: maximal tolerated intravesical dose, 6 mo high grade RLFS, 1 year RLFS Secondary: toxicity, high grade PFS at 30 d and 6 mo, PDL-1 expression in tumor and urine	December 2021
Nivolumab IV alone or with BMS-986205 ± BCG	NCT03519256	II	436	Primary: proportion of CIS with complete response up to 5 y, EFS, duration of complete response up to 5 y Secondary: PFS, incidence of adverse events, serious Adverse effects, death, and laboratory abnormalities	April 2023

Abbreviations: BCG, bacillus Calmette-Guerin; BCSS, bladder cancer–specific survival; CFS, cystectomy-free survival; CIS, carcinoma in situ; CRR, complete response rate; DFS, disease-free survival; DSS, disease-specific survival; EBRT, external beam radiotherapy; EFS, event-free survival; PD-1, programmed death-1; PDL-1, programmed death ligand-1; PFS, progression-free survival; QOL, quality of life; RFS, recurrence-free survival; RLFS, relapse-free survival rate.

cytokine therapy research that has primary focused on the effects of IL-2 and IL-15.[27] ALT-801, a recombinant humanized T-cell receptor–IL-2 fusion protein has shown immune responses and potential durable clinical activity in combination with gemcitabine in BCG-resistant NMIBC (NCT01625260) in a phase I setting and further update from this trial is awaited in the phase IIa setting.[29] ALT-803 is also being studied in a clinical trial setting following a report of beneficial effect in a 92-year-old patient who remained disease-free for 2.5 years after compassionate use.[30] ALT-803 is a complex of an IL-15 supera-gonist mutant and a dimeric IL-15 receptor a Su/Fc fusion protein, which is undergoing clinical trials for hematologic and solid malignancies and is the focus of a phase II, open-label, single-arm, multi-center study (NCT03022825) of intravesical BCG plus ALT-803 in patients with BCG-unresponsive high-grade NMIBC.[31] IL-15 is the most critical factor for the development, proliferation, and activation of natural killer and CD8 T cells and believed to be one of the most promising immunotherapeutic agents currently under study.[32] The primary end point is to assess complete response (absence of lesions on cystoscopy or negative, for cause, biopsies along with negative urine cytology) of carcinoma in situ at 6 months. It is estimated to enroll 160 patients and complete by September 2020.

Vaccines

Specific CD4[+] and CD8[+] T-cell immune response in solid tumors associated with carcinoembryonic antigen and mucin-1 antigen has been seen with the use of PANVAC, which is a pox viral vector-based vaccine.[33] Owing to this cellular immune response, a randomized, prospective phase I/II trial (NCT02015104) is using PANVAC with BCG to enhance and augment the BCG-induced T-cell response against bladder cancer cells expressing mucin-1 and/or carcinoembryonic antigen in patients who have failed at least 1 induction course of BCG. It has completed accrual of 32 patients and is intended to report on the primary outcome of improvement in disease-free survival with BCG + PANVAC compared with BCG alone.

A phase I/II trial (NCT02371447) is assessing the safety and efficacy of VPM1002BC, which is a genetically modified mycobacterium bovis BCG. The modification, which constitutes the insertion of the listeriolysin gene from *Listeria monocytogenes* and deletion of the urease C gene, is postulated to increase the immunogenicity of this BCG strain and decrease the side effects associated with intravesical instillation.[34] It has also completed accrual of 39 patients and is expected to report on the side effects as well as recurrence free rates in the bladder.

SUMMARY

The progressive incorporation of immunotherapy into the NMIBC setting is an exciting prospect given the initial promise shown in the early studies. It has the potential to revolutionize NMIBC treatment in patients with BCG-refractory disease to avoid radical cystectomy and preserve their bladder. Identifying the subgroup of patients who will respond to each of the different agents will be vital to make large leaps in this area.

REFERENCES

1. Babjuk M, Bohle A, Burger M, et al. EAU guidelines on non-muscle-invasive urothelial carcinoma of the bladder: update 2016. Eur Urol 2017;71:447–61.

2. Marigo I, Bosio E, Solito S, et al. Tumor-induced tolerance and immune suppression depend on the C/EBPbeta transcription factor. Immunity 2010;32: 790–802.

3. Eruslanov E, Neuberger M, Daurkin I, et al. Circulating and tumor-infiltrating myeloid cell subsets in patients with bladder cancer. Int J Cancer 2012 Mar 1;130(5):1109–19.

4. Droin N, Hendra JB, Ducoroy P, et al. Human defensins as cancer biomarkers and antitumour molecules. J Proteomics 2009;72:918–27.

5. Gunes M, Gecit I, Pirincci N, et al. Plasma human neutrophil proteins-1, -2, and -3 levels in patients with bladder cancer. J Cancer Res Clin Oncol 2013;139:195–9.

6. Vlahou A, Schellhammer PF, Mendrinos S, et al. Development of a novel proteomic approach for the detection of transitional cell carcinoma of the bladder in urine. Am J Pathol 2001;158: 1491–502.

7. Liu Y, Cao X. The origin and function of tumor-associated macrophages. Cell And Mol Immunol 2014;12:1.

8. Noy R, Pollard JW. Tumor-associated macrophages: from mechanisms to therapy. Immunity 2014;41: 49–61.

9. Lima L, Oliveira D, Tavares A, et al. The predominance of M2-polarized macrophages in the stroma of low-hypoxic bladder tumors is associated with BCG immunotherapy failure. Urol Oncol 2014;32: 449–57.

10. Ajili F, Kourda N, Darouiche A, et al. Prognostic value of tumor-associated macrophages count in human non-muscle-invasive bladder cancer treated by BCG immunotherapy. Ultrastruct Pathol 2013;37: 56–61.

11. Xu Z, Wang L, Tian J, et al. High expression of B7-H3 and CD163 in cancer tissues indicates malignant clinicopathological status and poor prognosis of patients with urothelial cell carcinoma of the bladder. Oncol Lett 2018;15:6519–26.

12. Hanada T, Nakagawa M, Emoto A, et al. Prognostic value of tumor-associated macrophage count in human bladder cancer. Int J Urol 2000;7:263–9.

13. Nishikawa H, Sakaguchi S. Regulatory T cells in tumor immunity. Int J Cancer 2010;127:759–67.

14. Chevalier MF, Schneider AK, Cesson V, et al. Conventional and PD-L1-expressing Regulatory T Cells are Enriched During BCG Therapy and may Limit its Efficacy. Eur Urol 2018;74:540–4.

15. Hashizume A, Umemoto S, Yokose T, et al. Enhanced expression of PD-L1 in non-muscle-invasive bladder cancer after treatment with Bacillus Calmette-Guerin. Oncotarget 2018;9:34066–78.

16. de Wit R, Kamat A, Nishiyama H, et al. 864OPembrolizumab for high-risk (HR) non–muscle invasive bladder cancer (NMIBC) unresponsive to bacillus

Calmette-Guérin (BCG): phase II KEYNOTE-057 trial. Ann Oncol 2018;29.

17. Balar AV, Kulkarni GS, Uchio EM, et al. Keynote 057: phase II trial of Pembrolizumab (Pembro) for patients (pts) with high-risk (HR) nonmuscle invasive bladder cancer (NMIBC) unresponsive to bacillus Calmette Guerin (BCG). J Clin Oncol 2019;37:350.

18. Wit RD, Kulkarni GS, Uchio EM, et al. Pembrolizumab (Pembro) for patients (pts) with high-risk (HR) non–muscle invasive bladder cancer (NMIBC) unresponsive to Bacillus Calmette-Guérin (BCG): updated follow-up from KEYNOTE-057. J Clin Oncol 2019;37:4530.

19. Powles T, Eder JP, Fine GD, et al. MPDL3280A (anti-PD-L1) treatment leads to clinical activity in metastatic bladder cancer. Nature 2014;515:558–62.

20. Rosenberg JE, Hoffman-Censits J, Powles T, et al. Atezolizumab in patients with locally advanced and metastatic urothelial carcinoma who have progressed following treatment with platinum-based chemotherapy: a single-arm, multicentre, phase 2 trial. Lancet 2016;387:1909–20.

21. Kamat AM, Bellmunt J, Choueiri TK, et al. KEYNOTE-057: phase 2 study of pembrolizumab for patients (pts) with Bacillus Calmette Guerin (BCG)-unresponsive, high-risk non-muscle-invasive bladder cancer (NMIBC). J Clin Oncol 2016;34. TPS4576-TPS.

22. Black PC, Catherine T, Lerner SP, et al. S1605: phase II trial of atezolizumab in BCG-unresponsive nonmuscle invasive bladder cancer. J Clin Oncol 2018;36:TPS527-TPS.

23. Hahn NM, Chang SS, Meng M, et al. A phase II, randomized study of nivolumab (nivo) or nivo plus BMS-986205 with or without intravesical Bacillus Calmette-Guerin (BCG) in BCG-unresponsive, high-risk, non-muscle invasive bladder cancer (NMIBC): CheckMate 9UT. J Clin Oncol 2019;37: TPS493-TPS.

24. Tabernero J, Luke JJ, Joshua AM, et al. BMS-986205, an indoleamine 2,3-dioxygenase 1 inhibitor (IDO1i), in combination with nivolumab (NIVO): updated safety across all tumor cohorts and efficacy in pts with advanced bladder cancer (advBC). J Clin Oncol 2018;36:4512.

25. Inman BA, Sebo TJ, Frigola X, et al. PD-L1 (B7-H1) expression by urothelial carcinoma of the bladder and BCG-induced granulomata: associations with localized stage progression. Cancer 2007;109: 1499–505.

26. Hudolin T, Mengus C, Coulot J, et al. Expression of indoleamine 2,3-dioxygenase gene is a feature of poorly differentiated non-muscle-invasive urothelial cell bladder carcinomas. Anticancer Res 2017;37: 1375–80.

27. Nykopp TK, Batista da Costa J, Mannas M, et al. Current clinical trials in non-muscle invasive bladder cancer. Curr Urol Rep 2018;19:101.

28. Rosenberg SA. IL-2: the first effective immunotherapy for human cancer. J Immunol 2014;192: 5451–8.

29. Sonpavde G, Rosser CJ, Pan C-x, et al. Phase I trial of ALT-801, a first-in-class T-cell receptor (TCR)-interleukin (IL)-2 fusion molecule, plus gemcitabine (G) for Bacillus Calmette Guerin (BCG)-resistant non-muscle-invasive bladder cancer (NMIBC). J Clin Oncol 2016;34:451.

30. Huang J, Schisler J, Wong HC, et al. Intravesical ALT-803 for BCG-unresponsive bladder cancer - a case report. Urol Case Rep 2017;14:15–7.

31. Chamie K, Salmasi A, Rosser CJ, et al. A multicenter clinical trial of intravesical BCG in combination with ALT-803 in patients with BCG-unresponsive non-muscle invasive bladder cancer. J Clin Oncol 2018;36:TPS544-TPS.

32. Waldmann TA. The biology of interleukin-2 and interleukin-15: implications for cancer therapy and vaccine design. Nat Rev Immunol 2006;6:595–601.

33. Gulley JL, Arlen PM, Tsang KY, et al. Pilot study of vaccination with recombinant CEA-MUC-1-TRICOM poxviral-based vaccines in patients with metastatic carcinoma. Clin Cancer Res 2008;14:3060–9.

34. Rentsch C, Bosshard P, Mayor G, et al. Results of the phase-I open-label clinical trial SAKK 06/14 assessing safety of intravesical instillation of the recombinant BCG VPM1002BC in patients with non-muscle invasive bladder cancer and previous failure to conventional BCG therapy. Eur Urol Suppl 2018; 17:e1050.

Role of Indoleamine-2,3-Dioxygenase Inhibitors in Salvage Therapy for Non-Muscle Invasive Bladder Cancer

Carissa E. Chu, MD[a], Sima P. Porten, MD, MPH[a],
Gary D. Grossfeld, MD, MPH[b], Maxwell V. Meng, MD[a],*

KEYWORDS

- IDO inhibitors • BCG-unresponsive • Non–muscle invasive bladder cancer

KEY POINTS

- The role of immunotherapy in the treatment of bladder cancer has spurred investigation into regulatory pathways of the immune system and subsequent interactions with tumor biology.
- Patients with BCG unresponsive non-muscle invasive bladder cancer have an unmet need for bladder sparing options, and existing therapies will require combination approaches to overcome immune escape.
- Indoleamine 2,3-dioxgenase 1 (IDO1) inhibitors are a class of small molecule drugs which have demonstrated efficacy in combination with existing immunotherapies in multiple types of advanced cancer, with increasing application in metastatic, muscle-invasive, and non-muscle Invasive bladder cancer.
- Manipulating the immune microenvironment with IDO1 inhibitors can increase sensitivity to existing therapies and augment the host response.

INTRODUCTION TO INDOLEAMINE-2,3-DIOXYGENASE 1 AND ROLE IN IMMUNOSUPPRESSION

Indoleamine-2,3-dioxygenase 1 (IDO1) is an intracellular immunoregulatory enzyme that serves as the first and rate-limiting step for the conversion of tryptophan to kynurenine (**Fig. 1**A).[1] The enzyme is highly expressed in the placenta and mucosa of the female genitourinary tract, lungs, and lymphoid organs, and its role has been implicated in maternal tolerance to fetus, allograft protection, and cancer progression.[2,3] This heme-dependent enzyme inserts an oxygen molecule across the 2 to 3 bond of the indole moiety of tryptophan.[4] Early observations in the 1950s showed elevated tryptophan catabolism in patients with bladder cancer, implicating the role of IDO1 in oncogenesis.[5] Subsequent studies have demonstrated that IDO1 mediates host immunosuppression due to the sensitivity of T cells to the presence of kynurenine and tryptophan deprivation, thereby driving immune escape.[6] Of note, a distinct pathway for the conversion of tryptophan to kynurenine by Trp 2,3-dioxygenase (TDO) also has been described, normally present in the liver and also found to have increased activity in tumor microenvironments.[7,8]

IDO1 activity is upregulated in tumor, stromal, and innate immune cells, where its expression is linked with shifting the tumor microenvironment

Disclosures: None.
[a] Department of Urology, University of California, San Francisco, 550 16th Street, 6th Floor, San Francisco, CA 94143, USA; [b] Bristol-Myers Squibb, 3401 Princeton Pike, Lawrenceville, New Jersey 08648, USA
* Corresponding author. Department of Urology, University of California, San Francisco, 550 16th Street, 6th Floor, San Francisco, CA 94143, USA.
E-mail address: max.meng@ucsf.edu

Urol Clin N Am 47 (2020) 111–118
https://doi.org/10.1016/j.ucl.2019.09.013

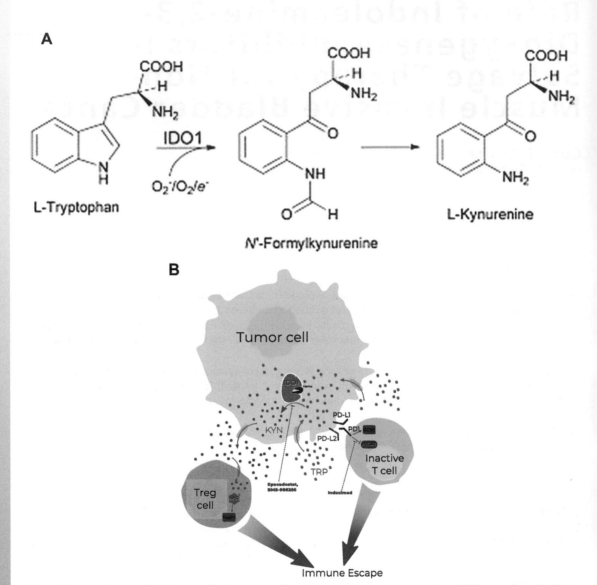

Fig. 1. (*A*) IDO1 is a rate-limiting step in the conversion of tryptophan to L-Kynurenine. (*B*) Tryptophan depletion by IDO1 activates T regulatory cells and inactivates T cells.

from immune activity to immune tolerance.[9] Several cancer cell types constitutively express IDO1, including melanoma, non-small cell cancer, renal cell carcinoma, bladder cancer, and cervical cancer.[10] Levels of kynurenine and kynurenine to tryptophan ratios are elevated in the serum of patients with cancer compared with healthy subjects.[11] By depleting tryptophan, IDO1 facilitates the suppression of CD8+ T effector and natural killer cells, generation and activation of CD4+ T regulatory and myeloid-derived suppressor cells, and promotion of tumor angiogenesis[12,13] (**Fig. 1**B). This mechanism occurs in concert with programmed cell death protein 1 (PD-1) pathways to induce immune quiescence. In fact, IDO1

expression increases after PD-1 blockade in patients with melanoma and renal cell carcinoma, suggesting a potential resistance mechanism of tumor cells to avoid immune detection.[14,15] In patients with bladder cancer failing Bacillus Calmette-Guerin (BCG) treatment, PD-L1 (ligand of PD-1) expression is associated with higher-grade tumors, infiltration by mononuclear cells, and BCG-induced granulomata.[16] In parallel, IDO1 expression is correlated with tumor size, grade, and stage in non–muscle invasive bladder cancer (NMIBC), and is present in 62% of bladder cancers.[17,18] By altering the tryptophan to kynurenine ratios, IDO1 can promote the tumor microenvironment. Downstream effector pathways of tryptophan depletion include repression of the mammalian target of rapamycin (mTOR) pathway and eukaryotic initiation factor 2 (eIF2) activation.[13] Increased kynurenine levels also activate the proinflammatory aryl-hydrocarbon receptor linked to carcinogenesis.[17,19,20] Thus, by altering the tryptophan to kynurenine ratio and by depleting tryptophan, IDO1 can trigger a robust response used by tumor cells to avoid immune surveillance.

DEVELOPMENT OF INDOLEAMINE-2,3-DIOXYGENASE 1 INHIBITORS IN CLINICAL TRIALS

Several factors support IDO1 and tryptophan catabolic pathways as promising therapeutic targets in bladder cancer. First, IDO1 is a small-molecule, single-chain catalytic enzyme with a well-defined biochemistry. Second, serum tryptophan measurements allow monitoring of IDO1 inhibition, making it an attractive target for drug development. Interest in the IDO1 enzyme as a target for cancer therapy began more than a decade ago, when preclinical models inhibiting IDO1 enhanced the efficacy of chemotherapy,[9] radiotherapy,[21] and immune checkpoint therapy[22] without a significant increase in adverse events (AEs).

In the past 5 years, 3 IDO1 inhibitors have reached at least phase II clinical trials and have demonstrated preliminary efficacy in patients with multiple types of advanced cancer. These IDO inhibitors are indoximod, epacadostat, and linrodostat mesylate (linrodostat; BMS-986205).

Other inhibitors are being tested in phase I trials, and additional patents have been filed (Roche, Merck) in the preclinical space (**Tables 1** and **2**).

INDOXIMOD

Indoximod inhibits mTORC1, a downstream effector of IDO1, and has progressed to phase III clinical trials. In an earlier phase II trial of 102 patients with heavily pretreated melanoma, indoximod with pembrolizumab achieved an overall response rate (ORR, including partial and complete responses) of 56% (19% complete response), which exceeds the 33% ORR of pembrolizumab monotherapy.[23] Given the inherent limitations of cross-trial comparisons between a single-arm phase II study, and a randomized controlled phase III study, and the limited sample size of this phase II trial compared with the much larger global phase III trial of nivolumab and ipilimumab in metastatic melanoma (CheckMate-067), these response rates appear to be comparable to the currently approved regimen of ipilimumab plus nivolumab but with potentially less immune-related toxicity.[24] In another phase II trial, patients with metastatic castrate-resistant prostate cancer treated with indoximod versus placebo after sipuleucel-T experienced greater than twofold increase in radiographic progression-free survival.[25] Other studies in breast cancer and acute myeloid leukemia are ongoing. NCT01792050 is a phase II clinical trial randomizing docetaxel plus indoximod versus docetaxel alone in patients with metastatic breast cancer with the primary endpoint of progression-free

Table 1
Current state of indoleamine-2,3-dioxygenase 1 inhibitors in development

Drug	Company	Mechanism	Trial Start	Program Status
Indoximod NLG-8186	NewLink	mTORC1 downstream activator	2008	Phase III
Epacadostat INCB024360	Incyte	Catalytic inhibitor	2012	Phase III
Linrodostat BMS 986205	BMS	Catalytic inhibitor	2015	Phase III
Navoximod NLG-919	NewLink	Catalytic inhibitor	2015	Phase IB
PF-06840003	Pfizer	Catalytic inhibitor	2016	Phase I
IOM2983	Merck	Unknown	Unknown	Preclinical
RG-70099	Roche	Dual IDO/TDO inhibitor	Unknown	Preclinical

Data from Prendergast GC, Malachowski WP, DuHadaway JB, Muller AJ. Discovery of IDO1 Inhibitors: From Bench to Bedside. Cancer Res. 2017;77(24):6795-6811. https://doi.org/10.1158/0008-5472.CAN-17-2285; and Gyulveszi G, Fischer C, Mirolo M, et al. Abstract LB-085: RG70099: A novel, highly potent dual IDO1/TDO inhibitor to reverse metabolic suppression of immune cells in the tumor micro-environment. *Cancer Res.* 2016;76(14 Supplement):LB-085-LB-085. https://doi.org/10.1158/1538-7445.AM2016-LB-085.

Table 2
Existing data on IDO1 inhibitors in patients with advanced bladder cancer

Drug	Patients, n	Objective Response Rate, %	Disease Control Rate, %	Clinical Trial	Phase	Comment
Linrodostat + nivolumab[39]	27	37	56	CA017-003	I/IIa	Anti-PD-1 monotherapy historically 15%–20% response rate
Epacadostat + pembrolizumab	40	35	53	ECHO-202/ KEYNOTE-037	I/II	Higher PD-L1 associated with higher overall response rate (64% vs 13%)

Abbreviations: IDO1, indoleamine-2,3-dioxygenase 1; PD-1, programmed cell death protein 1; PD-L1, ligand of PD-1.

survival; this trial is actively recruiting.[26] NCT02835729 is a phase II trial also in active recruitment, randomizing patients with acute myeloid leukemia to either indoximod or placebo while undergoing induction therapy with cytarabine and idarubicin; however, indoximod has not yet been studied in bladder cancer.

EPACADOSTAT

Epacadostat is a selective inhibitor against IDO1 that has been studied in several phase II trials. ECHO-202 was a multi-disease cohort of patients with advanced solid tumors treated with pembrolizumab and epacadostat, showing impressive early response rates of 33% to 58% across multiple tumor types (non-small cell lung cancer, renal cell carcinoma, endometrial adenocarcinoma, urothelial carcinoma, and squamous cell carcinoma of the head and neck), compared with 16% to 33% with pembrolizumab monotherapy.[27] By RECIST v1.1 criteria, 8 of 62 patients achieved complete response (5 patients with treatment-naïve melanoma, 3 patients with advanced and pretreated melanoma, urothelial cancer, and endometrial adenocarcinoma). Seventeen patients achieved partial response (treatment-naïve melanoma in 6 patients, non–small-cell lung cancer in 5 patients, and 2 patients each with renal cell carcinoma and urothelial carcinoma, and 1 patient each with endometrial adenocarcinoma, and head and neck cancer). Twenty-four percent of patients reported grade 3/4 AEs. ECHO-204 was a phase II study examining epacadostat in combination with nivolumab across multiple disease cohorts. Results included promising efficacy data with a 62% ORR across all patients, and a 65% ORR across 40 treatment-naïve patients. Grade 3 or

higher treatment-related adverse events were reported in 48% of patients treated at an epacadostat dose of 300 mg twice a day (most common AEs being rash and alanine aminotransferase increase), but in only 13% of patients treated at an epacadostat dose of 100 mg twice a day, which was the dosage that was selected for subsequent phase III studies.[28] In melanoma, epacadostat in combination with anti-PD-1 agents (pembrolizumab or nivolumab) achieved rates of response and disease control comparable to the approved combination of PD-1 and CTLA-4 antibodies but without similar rates of immune-mediated AEs and in a manner independent of PD-L1 levels.[25] Similarly promising results were found in patients with triple-negative breast, head and neck, endometrial, lung, renal, and urothelial cancers.[29,30] These findings were believed to be proof of concept that addition of epacadostat to checkpoint inhibitors could bolster response rates by synergizing with existing pharmacologic pathways.

Despite promising phase II data, a subsequent phase III trial in melanoma (ECHO-301/KEYNOTE-252) showed no improvement in progression-free survival with the epacadostat/pembrolizumab combination when compared with pembrolizumab alone. In 706 patients with unresectable or metastatic melanoma randomized to pembrolizumab with either epacadostat or placebo, there was no difference in median progression-free survival (4.7 vs 4.9 months, hazard ratio [HR] 1.0; 37% for both groups at 12 months), and overall survival was not expected to reach statistical significance based on results of interim analysis (HR 1.13; confidence interval 0.86–1.49; $P = .807$; 74% in both groups at 12 months). Median follow-up was 14 months and 72.5% of patients were PD-L1 positive.[31] It remains unclear whether the negative results from this trial were related to lack of efficacy, inadequate dosing of epacadostat, patient selection independent of biomarkers, or persistence of a parallel TDO pathway that mitigated the effects of the IDO1 inhibitor. As previously discussed, the TDO pathway has similar yet distinct downstream effects that may also deplete tryptophan and increase kynurenine. In melanoma, for example, IDO1 suppression alone may be insufficient to relieve the immunosuppressive effect of kynurenine.[8] The findings of ECHO-301/KEYNOTE-252 triggered the early termination of several other studies of IDO1 inhibitors, including linrodostat in melanoma and head and neck cancer (Bristol Meyers Squibb), indoximod in metastatic melanoma (Indigo 301, NewLink), and epacadostat (Incyte) in 6 other late-stage clinical trials.

LINRODOSTAT (BMS-986205): APPLICATION IN BLADDER CANCER

Linrodostat is a selective, potent, once-daily, oral IDO1 inhibitor that occupies the heme cofactor binding site, preventing activation of the IDO1 pathway to reduce kynurenine production.[32] Despite recent development challenges for IDO1 inhibitors, including the negative ECHO-301/KEYNOTE-252 study, the role of IDO inhibition in combination with anti-PD-L1 therapy in the treatment of bladder cancer appears promising. Phase II data from the combinations of pembrolizumab with epacadostat and nivolumab with linrodostat showed that in patients with advanced urothelial carcinoma who had received prior systemic treatment (cisplatinum or alternative), epacadostat and linrodostat potentially conferred additional antitumor activity when combined with checkpoint inhibitors compared with checkpoint inhibitors alone (ECHO-202/KEYNOTE-037 and CA017-003 studies, respectively).[33] In ECHO-202, a total of 40 patients with advanced bladder cancer refractory to prior platinum-based therapy demonstrated a 35% ORR (all partial responders) with a disease control rate (DCR: complete response, partial response, stable disease) of 57%. Progression-free survival and biomarker analyses are ongoing. The most common AEs were fatigue, rash, and increased amylase, and grade 3 or higher AEs occurred in 20% of patients.

In the phase I/IIa dose escalation study CA017-003, linrodostat in combination with nivolumab demonstrated clinical activity in 30 patients with advanced bladder cancer, all of whom had received at least 1 line of prior therapy. Eighty-three percent of these patients had baseline visceral metastases, including one-third with liver

metastasis, and 50% had PD-L1–positive tumors. The study demonstrated that the 100-mg dose of linrodostat was better tolerated than the 200-mg dose with similar efficacy. A 37% ORR and 56% DCR was observed in 27 patients with advanced bladder cancer who had not previously received immunotherapy. Median time to response was 7.8 weeks. The response rate was higher in PD-L1 positive versus PD-L1 negative tumors (50% vs 30% ORR, 64 vs 50% DCR). ORR was 30% in patients with baseline visceral metastases and 33% in patients with baseline liver metastases. Deep and durable reduction in tumor burden was observed in both PD-L1–positive and PD-L1–negative tumors, with some responses lasting beyond treatment discontinuation. Grade 3/4 treatment-related AEs occurred in 37% of all patients: 21% in patients treated with the 100-mg dose and 50% in patients treated with the 200-mg dose of linrodostat. Consequently, the 100-mg daily dose of linrodostat was established as the selected dose for phase II and III clinical trials moving forward.[32]

These results have laid the groundwork for 2 pivotal trials with linrodostat in bladder cancer. The phase II trial (CheckMate 9UT; NCT03519256) will investigate 4 different treatment regimens (nivolumab alone, nivolumab plus BCG, nivolumab plus linrodostat, or nivolumab plus linrodostat and BCG) in BCG-unresponsive, high-risk NMIBC (**Fig. 2**). Recruitment for this study is ongoing with an estimated goal of 480 enrolled patients. Follow-up will continue until disease recurrence/progression or for 5 years, and will include routine surveillance cystoscopy, cytology, and biopsy per American Urological Association and European Association of Urology guidelines. Primary endpoints include complete response rate (patients with carcinoma in situ (CIS)) and event-free survival (in all other patients). Secondary endpoints include progression-free survival as well as the safety and tolerability of the investigational treatments. Pharmacokinetics, potential predictive biomarkers, and changes in patient-reported outcome for quality of life also will be assessed.

The phase III CA017-078 trial (NCT 03661320) will study a perioperative treatment approach in patients with clinical stage T2-T4a, N0 muscle-invasive bladder cancer (MIBC) who are candidates for radical cystectomy. This randomized controlled study will enroll MIBC participants who are eligible to receive cisplatin-based chemotherapy with a creatinine clearance of 50 mL/min or greater. Participants will be randomized to 1 of 3 treatment arms: neoadjuvant chemotherapy (gemcitabine and cisplatin) followed by radical cystectomy, neoadjuvant nivolumab plus

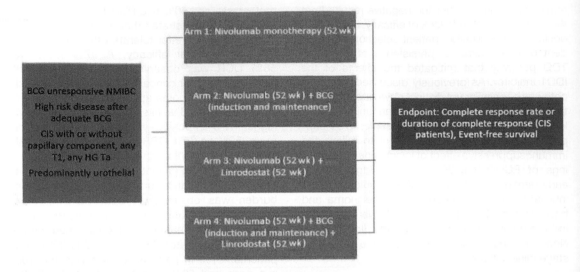

Fig. 2. CA209-9UT (NCT 03519256) phase II, open-label study assessing efficacy and safety of nivolumab ± linrodostat ± intravesical BCG via randomization of patients to 4 treatment arms. BCG, bacillus calmette-guerin; NMIBC, non-muscle invasive bladder cancer. (*Adapted from* Hahn NM, Chang SS, Meng M, et al. A phase II, randomized study of nivolumab (nivo) or nivo plus BMS-986205 with or without intravesical Bacillus Calmette-Guerin (BCG) in BCG-unresponsive, high-risk, non-muscle invasive bladder cancer (NMIBC): CheckMate 9UT. *J Clin Oncol.* 2019;37(7_suppl):TPS493-TPS493. https://doi.org/10.1200/JCO.2019.37.7_suppl.TPS493 with permission.)

chemotherapy followed by radical cystectomy and continued nivolumab, or neoadjuvant nivolumab plus linrodostat plus chemotherapy followed by radical cystectomy and continued nivolumab plus linrodostat. The primary endpoints for this study include pathologic complete response in the radical cystectomy specimen and event-free survival. Secondary endpoints include overall survival and safety.

RATIONALE FOR INDOLEAMINE-2,3-DIOXYGENASE USE AS SALVAGE TREATMENT IN NON–MUSCLE-INVASIVE BLADDER CANCER

Immunotherapy remains an attractive option for salvage therapy in BCG-unresponsive NMIBC, which continues to be a disease defined by recurrence and progression. Very few bladder-sparing options exist, and a variety of intravesical therapies, either as single agents or treatment combinations (valrubicin, gemcitabine, mitomycin, docetaxel, interferon) have been studied in the BCG-unresponsive population, with response rates ranging from 15% to 53%.[34] To date, there is insufficient evidence (small cohorts, short duration of follow-up) to incorporate these agents into current guidelines.[35]

The long-standing use of intravesical BCG as treatment for patients with NMIBC attests to the central role of the immune system in reducing recurrence and progression rates in this disease and supports evaluation of other immunotherapy strategies to overcome resistance to BCG. Higher-grade bladder cancers bear higher mutational burden[36] and are therefore antigenic.[37] This biology suggests that immune checkpoint inhibitors may be effective in patients at greater risk for recurrence and progression. Ongoing clinical trials are examining the use of checkpoint inhibitors in BCG-unresponsive, relapsing, and naive bladder cancer. Early results of KEYNOTE-057, a single-arm, open-label phase II study, showed that the use of pembrolizumab monotherapy in BCG-unresponsive CIS demonstrated a 38.8% complete response rate (defined as absence of any disease) at 3 months, and absence of progression to muscle-invasive disease with a median follow-up of 15.8 months (n=102).[38] However, the durability of response to pembrolizumab monotherapy remains a concern, with only 54% of CIS participants achieving a complete response (21% of the entire CIS cohort) maintaining this response after 9 months. A phase III study to evaluate pembrolizumab plus BCG versus BCG is now open to enrollment for BCG-relapsing disease (KEYNOTE-676). Two additional trials are open in BCG-naive disease: Potomac (NCT03528694) and Alban (NCT03799835).

As the management of NMIBC evolves, the need for well-tolerated, preferably oral agents with favorable safety profiles that can be combined with checkpoint inhibitors, such as IDO1 inhibitors, are needed to augment the efficacy and durability of checkpoint inhibitors in this disease that is characterized by recurrence and progression.

SUMMARY AND FUTURE PERSPECTIVES

The increase in the use of immunotherapy in the treatment of bladder cancer has spurred investigation into regulatory pathways that modulate the immune system. Enhancing clinical benefit and prolonging survival in more patients requires additional, combination approaches to overcome tumor evasion mechanisms. Manipulating the immune microenvironment can increase sensitivity to existing therapies and augment the host response, with the goal of preventing the immune escape of cancer.

Control of NMIBC requires leveraging existing knowledge about the immune response to cancer. The rise of immunotherapy in the management of advanced urothelial cancer supports a rationale for incorporating these therapies as bladder-sparing treatment in BCG-unresponsive NMIBC. The discovery of IDO1 has provided additional insight into the role of the local inflammatory state in tumor pathogenesis. IDO1 inhibitors may offer well-tolerated, oral regimens that can provide synergy to existing therapies.

ACKNOWLEDGMENTS

The authors acknowledge Sudarshan Srirangapatanam for creating **Fig. 1**B.

REFERENCES

1. Austin CJD, Kahlert J, Issa F, et al. The first indoleamine-2,3-dioxygenase-1 (IDO1) inhibitors containing carborane. Dalton Trans 2014;43(28):10719–24.
2. Mellor AL, Chandler P, Lee GK, et al. Indoleamine 2,3-dioxygenase, immunosuppression and pregnancy. J Reprod Immunol 2002;57(1–2):143–50. Available at: http://www.ncbi.nlm.nih.gov/pubmed/12385839. Accessed March 19, 2019.
3. Dai X, Zhu BT. Indoleamine 2,3-dioxygenase tissue distribution and cellular localization in mice: implications for its biological functions. J Histochem Cytochem 2010;58(1):17–28.
4. Geng J, Liu A. Heme-dependent dioxygenases in tryptophan oxidation. Arch Biochem Biophys 2014;544:18–26.
5. Boyland E, Williams D. The metabolism of tryptophan. 2. The metabolism of tryptophan in patients suffering from cancer of the bladder. Biochem J 1956;64(3):578–82. Available at: http://www.ncbi.nlm.nih.gov/pubmed/13373811. Accessed February 13, 2019.
6. Munn DH, Zhou M, Attwood JT, et al. Prevention of allogeneic fetal rejection by tryptophan catabolism. Science 1998;281(5380):1191–3. Available at: http://www.ncbi.nlm.nih.gov/pubmed/9712583. Accessed February 13, 2019.
7. Badawy AA-B. Kynurenine pathway of tryptophan metabolism: regulatory and functional aspects. Int J Tryptophan Res 2017;10. 1178646917691938.
8. Platten M, von Knebel Doeberitz N, Oezen I, et al. Cancer immunotherapy by targeting IDO1/TDO and their downstream effectors. Front Immunol 2014;5:673.
9. Muller AJ, DuHadaway JB, Donover PS, et al. Inhibition of indoleamine 2,3-dioxygenase, an immunoregulatory target of the cancer suppression gene Bin1, potentiates cancer chemotherapy. Nat Med 2005;11(3):312–9.
10. Uyttenhove C, Pilotte L, Théate I, et al. Evidence for a tumoral immune resistance mechanism based on tryptophan degradation by indoleamine 2,3-dioxygenase. Nat Med 2003;9(10):1269–74.
11. de Jong RA, Nijman HW, Boezen HM, et al. Serum tryptophan and kynurenine concentrations as parameters for indoleamine 2,3-Dioxygenase activity in patients with endometrial, ovarian, and vulvar cancer. Int J Gynecol Cancer 2011;21(7):1.
12. Mondal A, Smith C, DuHadaway JB, et al. IDO1 is an integral mediator of inflammatory neovascularization. EBioMedicine 2016;14:74–82.
13. Prendergast GC, Smith C, Thomas S, et al. Indoleamine 2,3-dioxygenase pathways of pathogenic inflammation and immune escape in cancer. Cancer Immunol Immunother 2014;63(7):721–35.
14. Urba WJ, Martín-Algarra S, Callahan M, et al. Abstract 2855: immunomodulatory activity of nivolumab monotherapy in patients with advanced melanoma. Cancer Res 2015;75(15 Supplement):2855.
15. Choueiri TK, Fishman MN, Escudier B, et al. Immunomodulatory activity of nivolumab in metastatic renal cell carcinoma. Clin Cancer Res 2016;22(22):5461–71.
16. Inman BA, Sebo TJ, Frigola X, et al. PD-L1 (B7-H1) expression by urothelial carcinoma of the bladder and BCG-induced granulomata. Cancer 2007;109(8):1499–505.
17. Moon YW, Hajjar J, Hwu P, et al. Targeting the indoleamine 2,3-dioxygenase pathway in cancer. J Immunother Cancer 2015;3(1):51.
18. Godin-Ethier J, Hanafi L-A, Piccirillo CA, et al. Indoleamine 2,3-dioxygenase expression in human

cancers: clinical and immunologic perspectives. Clin Cancer Res 2011;17(22):6985–91.

19. Prendergast GC, Malachowski WP, DuHadaway JB, et al. Discovery of IDO1 inhibitors: from bench to bedside. Cancer Res 2017;77(24):6795–811.

20. Spranger S, Koblish HK, Horton B, et al. Mechanism of tumor rejection with doublets of CTLA-4, PD-1/PD-L1, or IDO blockade involves restored IL-2 production and proliferation of CD8+ T cells directly within the tumor microenvironment. J Immunother Cancer 2014;2(1):3.

21. Monjazeb AM, Kent MS, Grossenbacher SK, et al. Blocking indolamine-2,3-dioxygenase rebound immune suppression boosts antitumor effects of radio-immunotherapy in murine models and spontaneous canine malignancies. Clin Cancer Res 2016; 22(17):4328–40.

22. Holmgaard RB, Zamarin D, Munn DH, et al. Indoleamine 2,3-dioxygenase is a critical resistance mechanism in antitumor T cell immunotherapy targeting CTLA-4. J Exp Med 2013;210(7):1389–402.

23. Zakharia Y, Rixe O, Ward JH, et al. Phase 2 trial of the IDO pathway inhibitor indoximod plus checkpoint inhibition for the treatment of patients with advanced melanoma. J Clin Oncol 2018; 36(15_suppl):9512.

24. Wolchok JD, Chiarion-Sileni V, Gonzalez R, et al. Overall survival with combined nivolumab and ipilimumab in advanced melanoma. N Engl J Med 2017;377(14):1345–56.

25. Jha GG, Gupta S, Tagawa ST, et al. A phase II randomized, double-blind study of sipuleucel-T followed by IDO pathway inhibitor, indoximod, or placebo in the treatment of patients with metastatic castration resistant prostate cancer (mCRPC). J Clin Oncol 2017;35(15_suppl):3066.

26. Soliman HH, Minton SE, Ismail-Khan R, et al. A phase 2 study of docetaxel in combination with indoximod in metastatic breast cancer. J Clin Oncol 2014;32(15_suppl):TPS3124.

27. Gangadhar TC, Schneider BJ, Bauer TM, et al. Efficacy and safety of epacadostat plus pembrolizumab treatment of NSCLC: preliminary phase I/II results of ECHO-202/KEYNOTE-037. J Clin Oncol 2017;35(15_suppl):9014.

28. Daud A, Saleh MN, Hu J, et al. Epacadostat plus nivolumab for advanced melanoma: updated phase 2 results of the ECHO-204 study. J Clin Oncol 2018; 36(15_suppl):9511.

29. Rose S. Epacadostat shows value in two SCCHN trials. Cancer Discov 2017;7(9):OF2.

30. Mitchell TC, Hamid O, Smith DC, et al. Epacadostat plus pembrolizumab in patients with advanced solid tumors: phase i results from a multicenter, open-label phase I/II Trial (ECHO-202/KEYNOTE-037). J Clin Oncol 2018. https://doi.org/10.1200/JCO.2018.78.9602. JCO2018789602.

31. Long GV, Dummer R, Hamid O, et al. Epacadostat (E) plus pembrolizumab (P) versus pembrolizumab alone in patients (pts) with unresectable or metastatic melanoma: results of the phase 3 ECHO-301/KEYNOTE-252 study. J Clin Oncol 2018;36(15_suppl):108.

32. Tabernero J, Luke JJ, Joshua AM, et al. BMS-986205, an indoleamine 2,3-dioxygenase 1 inhibitor (IDO1i), in combination with nivolumab (NIVO): updated safety across all tumor cohorts and efficacy in pts with advanced bladder cancer (advBC). J Clin Oncol 2018;36(15_suppl):4512.

33. Smith DC, Gajewski T, Hamid O, et al. Epacadostat plus pembrolizumab in patients with advanced urothelial carcinoma: preliminary phase I/II results of ECHO-202/KEYNOTE-037. J Clin Oncol 2017; 35(15_suppl):4503.

34. Kamat AM, Sylvester RJ, Böhle A, et al. Definitions, end points, and clinical trial designs for non-muscle-invasive bladder cancer: recommendations from the International Bladder Cancer Group. J Clin Oncol 2016;34(16):1935–44.

35. Peyton CC, Chipollini J, Azizi M, et al. Updates on the use of intravesical therapies for non-muscle invasive bladder cancer: how, when and what. World J Urol 2018;1–13. https://doi.org/10.1007/s00345-018-2591-1.

36. Pietzak EJ, Bagrodia A, Cha EK, et al. Next-generation sequencing of nonmuscle invasive bladder cancer reveals potential biomarkers and rational therapeutic targets. Eur Urol 2017;72(6):952–9.

37. Schumacher TN, Schreiber RD. Neoantigens in cancer immunotherapy. Science 2015;348(6230):69–74.

38. Balar AV, Kulkarni GS, Uchio EM, et al. Keynote 057: Phase II trial of Pembrolizumab (pembro) for patients (pts) with high-risk (HR) nonmuscle invasive bladder cancer (NMIBC) unresponsive to bacillus calmette-guérin (BCG). J Clin Oncol 2019; 37(7_suppl):350. https://doi.org/10.1200/JCO.2019.37.7_suppl.350.

39. Luke JJ, Gelmon K, Pachynski RK, et al. Preliminary antitumor and immunomodulatory activity of BMS-986205, an optimized indoleamine 2, 3-dioxygenase 1 (IDO1) inhibitor, in combination with nivolumab in patients with advanced cancers. National Harbor, MD: SITC; 2017. Abstract O41.

Salvage Therapy for Non–muscle-invasive Bladder Cancer: Novel Intravesical Agents

Dunia Khaled, MD[a], John Taylor, MD[b], Jeffrey Holzbeierlein, MD[a],*

KEYWORDS

- Non–muscle-invasive bladder cancer • BCG failure • Novel agents • Intravesical therapy

KEY POINTS

- Novel intravesical therapies have modest response rates to date.
- Combination intravesical chemotherapies, new modes of delivery, and immunotherapy hold promise.
- Results of the various clinical trials are presented.

INTRODUCTION

Three-quarters of newly diagnosed urothelial cancers are non–muscle-invasive bladder cancer (NMIBC). Unfortunately, rates of recurrence and progression remain high, with 8% having progression at 1 year and even a mortality rate of 1%.[1] High-risk NMIBCs, such as those with high-grade T1 tumors and concomitant carcinoma in situ (CIS), have even higher progression rates of approximately 30%. The risk of waiting for progression is demonstrated by patients with recurrent T1 disease who fail bacillus Calmette-Guerin (BCG) and progress and have a delay in cystectomy. A study by Herr and Sogani[2] demonstrated that patients who have an early cystectomy have significantly higher disease-specific survival as compared with those who undergo surgery beyond 2 years (92% vs 56%).

The standard of care for high-risk NMIBC is induction and maintenance intravesical instillation BCG.[2] Despite this, approximately 37% to 45%, of patients treated over a 2-year span with BCG will fail. Because of the lack of alternative conservative treatments, radical cystectomy (RC) is recommended and stands as the standard of care

when recurrence occurs.[3] The American Urological Association Guidelines specifically recommend that RC should be performed in patients with persistent high-grade disease or recurrence within 6 months of receiving at least 2 courses of intravesical BCG (at least 5 of 6 induction and at least 2 of 3 maintenance doses of BCG) and patients with T1 high-grade disease at the first evaluation following induction BCG (at least 5 of 6 doses).[3] Although RC remains the standard of care in these patients, national practice patterns suggest that many patients are not getting a cystectomy when indicated, likely due to age, comorbidities, and/or desire to avoid such surgery.[4]

There are no established, effective intravesical therapies available for patients with tumor recurrence after BCG to compete with RC; however, the well-selected patient may be offered conservative bladder-sparing therapies, and several new options are emerging. To date, the only Food and Drug Administration (FDA)-approved agent for BCG-refractory patients with CIS is intravesical valrubicin, although long-term outcomes are poor compared with those of RC. The aim of this study was to review the current literature regarding salvage therapies for patients with

Disclosure Statement: The authors have nothing to disclose.
a Department of Urology, University of Kansas Medical Center, 3901 Rainbow Boulevard, Mail Stop 3016, Kansas City, KS 66160, USA; b Department of Urology, University of Kansas Medical Center, Kansas City, KS, USA
* Corresponding author.
E-mail address: jholzbeierlein@kumc.edu

Urol Clin N Am 47 (2020) 119–128
https://doi.org/10.1016/j.ucl.2019.09.014
0094-0143/20/© 2019 Elsevier Inc. All rights reserved.

BCG failure, with a particular focus on recently developed treatments and ongoing trials. Alternative treatments for patients with NMIBC are under investigation to augment or replace BCG immunotherapy, including combination therapies with well-known cytotoxic intravesical chemotherapies, novel delivery techniques, cytokine therapy, chemoradiation, chemohyperthermia, viral gene therapy, targeted therapy, vaccination strategies, checkpoint inhibitors, and systemic immunotherapy (**Fig. 1**).

SALVAGE THERAPIES TO DATE
Repeat Bacillus Calmette-Guerin

Select patients may undergo repeat BCG induction. In the setting of CIS or positive cytology at 3 months after induction, repeat induction can achieve complete response (CR) in more than 50% of cases based on meta-analysis of 9 randomized trials including 700 patients over a median follow-up of 3.6 years.[5] Patients with a high-grade Ta tumor or CIS at 3 months after induction may also undergo repeat induction with reevaluation at 6 months.[5] In the setting of a

BCG relapse, a second induction course of BCG may be given if no maintenance was given; in an older cohort, this has been associated with a 40% response rate.[6] However, more than 2 courses of induction BCG are not recommended because of the greatly reduced chance of success (<20%), coupled with increased likelihood of tumor progression (30%) and metastasis (50%).[7] Finally, patients with late BCG relapse, recurrence more than 1 year after BCG treatments, have been shown to have similar cancer-free rates as BCG-naïve patients and reinduction BCG should be considered.[6,7] As discussed previously, although reinduction BCG is appropriate for these select BCG-resistant and BCG-relapsing disease states, data to support its use in BCG-refractory or recurrent T1 disease is insufficient.

Overall, as one of the earliest effective immunotherapies, intravesical BCG has been embraced as the standard of care for NMIBC for more than 3 decades and is appropriate to use in select salvage settings; however, it is not without its inherent challenges. BCG is dependent on the growth of the mycobacterium under controlled circumstances, which can be achieved by a limited

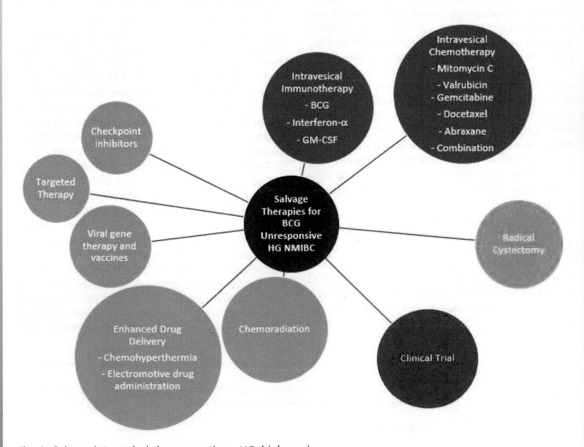

Fig. 1. Salvage intravesical therapy options. HG, high grade.

number of manufacturers, and as such, BCG is susceptible to shortages. Furthermore, for those unwilling or unable to undergo induction or maintenance BCG secondary to BCG side effects or for those with an unwillingness or inability to undergo cystectomy, alternative treatment strategies are required.

Intravesical Chemotherapy: Mitomycin C

Mitomycin C (MMC) is an antineoplastic antibiotic that cross-links DNA preventing synthesis. In addition, MMC is a desiccant of urothelial tissue allowing for increased permeability to intravesical agents. It has been most commonly used as a single instillation administered at the time of transurethral resection of a bladder tumor, particularly for low-grade disease. The role of MMC alone as a salvage therapy in high-risk NMIBC has not been fully elucidated in a randomized trial, although some inferential conclusions may be made. Malmström and colleagues[8] enrolled 261 patients including patients with primary high-risk and recurrent Ta and T1 bladder cancer. According to the protocol, crossover treatment was administered to 21 patients who changed from BCG to second-line MMC. Of this group, only 4 (19%) had recurrence-free survival (RFS) at 3 years.

Intravesical Chemotherapy: Valrubicin

Valrubicin is a semisynthetic anthracycline. Currently, valrubicin is the only FDA-approved therapy for BCG-refractory CIS based on a single-arm trial of 90 patients who had CIS or high-grade Ta and T1 disease; 99% of whom who had failed at least 2 cycles of prior intravesical therapy, most commonly BCG.[9] In this cohort, 18% to 21% had a CR at 6 months and 8% at 24 months, with a median follow-up of 30 months. RC was completed in 56% of the patients, and 15% had pT3 or greater staging at time of cystectomy. All cancer-specific deaths were in patients who did not undergo cystectomy or experienced a CR. Updated reports of the original study were reported along with a reports from a second single-arm study of valrubicin for BCG-refractory CIS, which included 80 BCG-refractory and BCG-intolerant patients (39% of whom had received ≥2 courses of BCG and 11% of whom had received ≥3 courses of BCG).[10] In this study, the CR was 18% for both groups.

Since the reintroduction of valrubicin in 2009, a contemporary cohort of 100 patients who completed salvage valrubicin treatment (51.3% with CIS alone) were retrospectively reviewed. RFS was 51.6% at 3 months, 30.4% at 6 months, and 16.4% at 12 months,[11] consistent with previous clinical trial findings. Overall, despite its FDA approval, valrubicin has very low response rates, and is a suboptimal salvage therapy in the setting of BCG failure. This has been one of the major impetuses for trials in this disease space.

Intravesical Chemotherapy: Gemcitabine

Gemcitabine is a pyrimidine analog that blocks DNA replication leading to apoptosis of cancer cells that has been extensively studied for salvage therapy. As a nonvesicant chemotherapy, it does not cause direct tissue injury when applied intravesically.

A phase II trial of 30 patients who were BCG refractory or BCG intolerant (20 with ≥2 prior BCG courses) who refused cystectomy were given 2 courses of intravesical gemcitabine twice weekly for 3 weeks.[12] Dalbagni and colleagues[12] reported a disease-free rate of 21% at 12 months. A multicenter phase II Southwest Oncology Group study evaluated single-agent intravesical gemcitabine given as a 6-week induction course followed by monthly maintenance for a year in high-risk patients (86% of the cohort) who had received ≥2 prior BCG courses.[13] They found RFS rates of 28% at 1 year and 21% at 2 years after therapy.[13] Two patients had disease progression, and 32% underwent cystectomy, although only 6% of those were found to have pT2 disease or higher in the pathologic specimen.

The true efficacy of gemcitabine in the pure BCG-refractory cohort is not known based on these studies, as these study populations were heterogeneous. However, direct comparisons have been made with known existing therapies. Di Lorenzo and colleagues[14] directly compared gemcitabine (GC) with BCG and demonstrated that, after failure of single BCG course, patients with high risk NMIBC have significantly better (52.3% vs 87.5%) disease recurrence if they were given intravesical gemcitabine induction with maintenance versus repeat BCG. Progression was greater than 35% in both groups, likely owing to the greater than 70% of patients with T1 disease in this very high-risk cohort. Overall, these data suggest GC may be an improved option relative to BCG alone. Similarly, when compared with MMC, gemcitabine has superior disease-free survival and lower toxicity.[15]

Intravesical Chemotherapy: Taxanes

Docetaxel is a microtubule depolymerization inhibitor with antimitotic tumor activity. In a phase II trial of 54 patients with BCG-refractory disease (28 who received BCG alone, 26 who received BCG and interferon [IFN]α, and 12 who additionally received MMC), a 6-week induction course of weekly intravesical docetaxel with monthly maintenance was administered.[16] A CR rate was achieved in 59%. At 1 year and 3 years, the RFS rates were 40% and 25%, respectively. An RC was performed in 24% at a median 24-month follow-up, and 4 of the 17 specimens showed progression to muscle-invasive disease.

Abraxane, a nanoparticle albumin-bound version of paclitaxel that is thought to have increased bioavailability when compared with docetaxel, has also been studied in a phase II trial.[17] At 1 year, RFS was 36% in a similar cohort of 28 patients.

NOVEL SALVAGE AGENTS
Combination Therapies

Combination chemotherapy regimens have been explored similar to multi-agent intravenous therapy, and these have been described in detail. Although the combination of drugs may result in increased toxicity, it may be advantageous to combine non-desiccant cytotoxic therapeutic drugs, such as gemcitabine and docetaxel, with desiccant drugs, such as mitomycin, to enable both drugs to be administered sequentially and take advantage of multiple mechanisms of action.

Steinberg and colleagues[1] first described sequential intravesical GC and docetaxel. They demonstrated 66% success at first surveillance, 54% at 1 year, and 34% at 2 years. Of those who proceeded to cystectomy, the findings were of favorable pathology without lymph node involvement or positive surgical margins.

Combination intravesical therapies with MMC also have been examined. Cockerill and colleagues[18] retrospectively reviewed a small cohort given sequential GC and MMC weekly. Durable responses were seen in 37% at 22.1 months of follow-up. In another multi-institutional series of 47 patients,[19] an initial CR of 68% was seen, with RFS rates of 48% at 1 year and 38% at 2 years posttreatment.[18,19]

These small trials suggest that couplet and combination therapies may demonstrate improved efficacy and warrant further investigation. Novel drug combinations are currently being explored and multiple combinations are in phase 1 trial testing. For example, NCT02202772 is testing intravesical gemcitabine, cabazitaxel, and cisplatin in BCG-unresponsive patients.

Granulocyte-Macrophage Colony-Stimulating Factor

Incomplete immunostimulation has been proposed as a possible etiology for BCG failure. Granulocyte-macrophage colony-stimulating factor (GM-CSF) has been identified as a stimulatory cytokine in the proinflammatory BCG pathway.[20] Therefore, its addition to intravesical treatment is thought to augment the proinflammatory response. Steinberg and colleagues[21] performed a retrospective review of BCG-failure patients who were given quadruple immunotherapy (reduced dose BCG, IFNα, interleukin [IL]-2, and GM-CSF). Treatment success was 53% at 2 years. Of those who underwent cystectomy, no patients had positive surgical margins or positive lymph nodes. This is promising, as it implies there is a window between BCG failure during which time salvage therapies may be explored without compromising curative surgery.

Chemoradiation

Although historically reserved for the muscle-invasive bladder cancer setting, chemoradiation has been explored in the NMIBC setting. Weiss and colleagues[22] published their experience at a single institution of 141 patients with high-risk T1 bladder cancer. They performed a debulking transurethral resection followed by pelvic (50.4 Gy) and bladder (55.8 Gy) radiation and cisplatin or carboplatin. CR was found to be 88%, with 5-year and 10-year progression rates of 19% and 30%, respectively. Although this was a primary treatment for NMIBC (not in a BCG-refractory cohort) and may not directly apply to the salvage setting, the results are promising.

A small cohort of 18 patients who had T1 tumors and progressed to T2 disease despite BCG therapy were treated with chemoradiotherapy, and at the median follow-up of 7 years, 54% were alive without cystectomy, without metastatic disease, and without muscle-invasive recurrence.[23] The investigators suggest this may be a viable option in the setting of T1 tumors that recur after BCG. However, in the setting of CIS, radiotherapy is not appropriate, as there is a high risk of bladder tumor recurrence.[24]

Currently ongoing is a nonrandomized phase II trial in patients with high-grade NMIBC after BCG failure giving either 61.2 Gy of radiation therapy with cisplatin after maximal transurethral resection or radiation therapy with 5-fluorouracil or MMC (NCT00981656). The primary endpoint is cystectomy-free survival. Based on the results, trimodal therapy may become an option for selected patients with BCG failure who are unfit for RC.

The National Cancer Institute's Clinical Trials planning meeting on novel therapeutics for NMIBC highlights that although the data are limited for the role of radiation therapy in NMIBC, radiation therapy is known to have direct impacts on immune-mediated effects, including chemotherapy or immune checkpoint inhibitors and should be explored.[25]

Novel Drug Administration: Chemohyperthermia

Chemohyperthermia (C-HT) is the combination of intravesical chemotherapy with hyperthermia of the intravesical agent. Hyperthermia raises temperatures within the bladder to 40 to 44°C. The heat alters intracellular metabolism resulting in DNA damage and induced apoptosis. There is also an increase in blood perfusion and cell permeability allowing for increased uptake of intravesical agents.[26,27] Currently, the European Association of Urology guidelines on C-HT holds a grade B recommendation for patients with BCG failure who are ineligible for RC.[28]

Hyperthermia can be achieved by intravesical microwave-induced heating via a radiofrequency-emitting antenna in a catheter, conductive heating via externally heated chemotherapy fluid, or locoregionally via external radiofrequency antennas.[26] Synergo is an FDA-approved computerized C-HT administration system and is the most widely used and studied.[26] COMBAT BRS is a recirculating system that externally heats MMC via conductive aluminum heating, which is then delivered via a 3-way urethral catheter.[26] BSD-200 is an FDA-approved system that uses electromagnetic waves to induce heat. Computerized tomography is used to plan treatment and localized temperature probes within the rectum and bladder, while externally located antenna pairs deliver radiofrequency waves to the pelvis.[26]

Optimized delivery strategies for MMC have been well studied and reviewed.[29] Routine clinical practice includes increased drug concentration to 40 mg MMC in 20 mL saline solution, alkalization of urine with oral sodium bicarbonate preoperatively, decreased drug dilution with fluid restriction, confirmation of an empty bladder with ultrasonography after catheterization, and a 2-hour dwell time. Although multiple studies have been published with addition of C-HT for optimization, most include patients with no prior intravesical therapies alongside chemotherapy and BCG treatments. It also must be mentioned that MMC displays greater toxicity under increased temperature.[30]

Colombo and colleagues[31] completed a small, multicenter prospective randomized control trial using Synergo comparing C-HT with MMC versus conventional MMC administration in 83 patients with high-risk primary NMIBC (35%–39% of the cohort) or recurrent NMIBC (approximately 60%–

65% of the cohort). After a 24-month median follow-up, recurrence rate in the C-HT with the MMC group was 17.1% versus 57.5% with the MMC group alone. Although promising, this cohort did include primary treatment, and these data have not been replicated.

Other retrospective analyses exist of C-HT with MMC in a BCG-refractory cohort. These have variable results. One-year and 2-year RFS of 85% and 56% respectively have been reported,[32] and these are lower in BCG-refractory patients with CIS with 1-year and 2-year recurrence rates at 23% and 41%, respectively.[33] In another CIS cohort, an initial response rate to hyperthermia was reported with MMC of 92% at 1 year and 50% at 2 years.[34] There was no difference in response rates seen in the subgroup of 34 BCG-failure patients.

Overall, recurrence rates are variable for patients with prior BCG failure after C-HT. Data on progression are scarce, and longer follow-up is needed. But these study designs portend slow accrual. For example, a direct comparison of MMC versus BCG in intermediate-risk and high-risk NMIBC (NCT00384891) was terminated early for slow accrual.

Novel Drug Administration: Electromotive Administration

Electromotive administration (EMDA) accelerates drug delivery through bladder mucosa by application of an electric field. The lower abdomen is grounded with electrodes and a transurethral catheter serves as the active electrode. Electrokinetic mechanisms of iontophoresis, electroosmosis, electrophoresis, and electroporation are suggested.[35] Current data have focused on its use as primary treatment. Racioppi and colleagues[36] carried out a single-arm phase II study of 26 BCG-refractory patients with 3-year follow-up. EMDA-MMC was given as induction with maintenance and surveilled with systemic mapping biopsies. At the end of follow-up, 61.5% of patients were able to preserve their bladders. The 23.1% who had recurrent high-grade disease and 15.4% who progressed to muscle-invasive disease underwent cystectomy. Disease-free states were lowest (25%) for patients with both high-grade disease and CIS and highest for Ta-only recurrence (75%).

Novel Drug Administration: Viral Gene Therapy and Vaccines

A nonreplicating adenovirus that is able to infect bladder urothelium and contains transgenes is thought to enhance cytotoxic immune response to tumor serves as the basis of viral gene therapy.

CG00700 was found in a phase I and II trial of BCG-refractory and BCG-relapsing disease to have 49% response rate at 10.4 months.[37,38]

Instiladrin (rAd-IFNα/Syn3) is an adenovirus encoding the human IFNα 2b transgene along with Syn3, a surfactant that enhances adenoviral transduction into the urothelium. In phase I and phase II trials of BCG-unresponsive patients, a CR of 36% was noted at 12 months.[39,40] A single-arm phase III trial (NCT02773849) is pending.

PANVAC is a poxviral vaccine that encodes genes for tumor-associated mucin-1 and carci-noembryonic antigens as well as T-cell costimula-tory molecules. NCT02015104 is a phase II trial of BCG with PANVAC in patients having failed 1 course of BCG induction.

Data from a single-arm phase Ib/II trial of BCG-refractory and BCG-relapsing patients showed CR >12 months in 2 of 6 patients on ALT-801, a re-combinant fusion protein of IL-2 plus a T-cell re-ceptor domain that recognizes human p53 antigen on cancer cells.[41] A review of the agents discussed, and their efficacy, is shown in **Tables 1** and **2**.

TARGETED THERAPY

VB4-845 (Vicinium) is an intravesical therapy that binds to epithelial cell adhesion molecule (EpCAM), an antibody overexpressed in cancer cells. This binding triggers internalization and up-take of a pseudomonal exotoxin causing cell death. In phase I studies including BCG-intolerant and BG-relapsing disease, RFS was 39% at 3 months.[42] A single-arm phase III trial (NCT02449239) is ongoing.

Everolimus, a mammalian target of rapamycin inhibitor, is being investigated with intravesical GC in a phase I/II trial of BCG-intolerant, BCG-un-responsive, and BCG-relapsing patients (NCT01259063).

The results of a tyrosine kinase inhibitor, oral sunitinib, in patients with recurrent NMIBC after BCG are pending. This trial (NCT01118351) has completed accrual and is pending report of findings.

NOVEL AGENTS: BENCH TO BEDSIDE

Based on discoveries in the laboratory leading to the identification of multiple pathways with poten-tially targetable lead candidates, novel therapies are entering into clinical trials. Although early in the pipeline, the following drugs show promise in their treatment of NMIBC as well as offering poten-tially novel methods of administration.

Fosciclopirox (CPX-POM)

Ciclopirox (CPX) is an FDA-approved antifungal agent with reported in vitro and in vivo anticancer activity. CPX activity in cancer is related to its iron chelation properties as well as its effect on pathways inclusive of notch, hedgehog, and wnt/b-catenin. However, its clinical utility is limited due to poor oral bioavailability, gastrointestinal toxicity, and poor water solubility.

Ciclopirox Prodrug (CPX-POM) is an investiga-tional small-molecule, novel anticancer agent being developed for the treatment of NMIBC. CPX-POM is fully soluble and intravenous admin-istration selectively delivers the active metabolite CPX, and its major inactive glucuronide metabolite (CPX-G), to the entire urinary tract at concentra-tions exceeding in vitro half maximal inhibitory concentration values. In addition, dramatically elevated ß-glucuronidase activity was observed in urine obtained from patients with NMIBC, suffi-cient to hydrolyze CPX-G resulting in reactivation of CPX within the urinary tract with possibility for potentiating effects.

In vitro data show that CPX inhibits cell prolifer-ation, colony formation, and bladdosphere forma-tion in high-grade bladder cancer cell lines.[43] Cell cycle arrest at the S and G0/G1 phases as well as apoptotic cell death were also noted. Preclinical in vivo data in the validated chemical carcinogen

Table 1 BCG failure definitions	
Types of BCG Failure	
BCG intolerance	Inability to received adequate BCG[a] secondary to toxicity
BCG refractory	HG disease at 6 mo despite adequate BCG OR stage or grade progression at 3 mo of BCG
BCG relapsing	HG recurrence at 6 mo despite adequate BCG OR stage or grade progression at 3 mo of BCG
BCG unresponsive	Includes *BCG-refractory* and *BCG-relapsing* groups, at highest risk of recurrence and progression

Abbreviations: BCG, Bacillus Calmette-Guerin; HG, high grade.
[a] Adequate BCG = at least induction (with minimum 5 of 6 instillations) and at least 1 maintenance (with mini-mum 2 of 3 instillations) in a 6-month period.

Table 2
Summary disease-free and recurrence-free survival for current salvage therapies

Treatment	RFS	
Standard of care: radical cystectomy	5-y CSS 80%	
Target rates based on consensus panels	50% RFS at 6 mo, 30% at 12 mo, 25% at 18 mo	
Gemcitabine	21%–28% RFS at 12 mo	21% RFS at 24 mo
Docetaxel	40% RFS at 12 mo	
Valrubicin	18%–21% RFS at 6 mo	16% RFS at 12 mo
Abraxane	36% RFS at 12 mo	
Gemcitabine/Docetaxel	54% RFS at 12 mo	34% RFS at 24 mo
Gemcitabine/MMC	48% RFS at 12 mo	38% RFS at 24 mo
BCG/INFα		45% RFS at 24 mo
BCG/INFα/IL-2/GM-CSF	55% RFS at 12 mo	53% RFS at 24 mo
Chemohyperthermia	Range 44–92 RFS at 12 mo	Range 50%–68.9% RFS at 24 mo
Chemoradiation		54% RFS at 24 mo
EMDA	53% RFS at 3 mo	58% RFS at 6 mo

Abbreviations: BCG, Bacillus Calmette-Guerin; CSS, cancer-specific survival; EMDA, electromotive drug administration; GM-CSF, granulocyte-macrophage colony-stimulating factor; HG, high grade; IL-2, interleukin-2; INFα, interferon α; MMC, mitomycin C; RFS, recurrence-free survival.

BBN mouse model showed significant decreases in bladder weight, a clear migration to lower-stage tumors, and dose-dependent reduction in Ki67 staining.[44] In addition, dose-dependent decreases in Notch 1, Presenilin 1, and Hey 1 were noted in bladder cancer tissues from CPX-POM–treated animals.

The FDA approved CPX-POM for Investigational New Drug status and the first-in-human US multicenter, phase I, dose-escalation study to evaluate safety, dose tolerance, pharmacokinetics, and pharmacodynamics (NCT03348514) in patients with unselected advanced solid tumors. This phase I trial was recently completed and the results published.[45] Based on this trial, no significant dose-limiting adverse events were noted, and expansion cohorts are planned to begin in patients with NMIBC.

MACROPHAGE MIGRATION INHIBITORY FACTOR

Macrophage migration inhibitory factor (MIF) is a pleiotropic inflammatory cytokine with many identified protumorigenic properties.[46] MIF activates many proliferative pathways, interferes with both the p53 and pRb tumor suppressor pathways, and increases angiogenesis as well as cellular migration/invasion.[46] As such, inhibition of MIF with monoclonal antibodies and small molecules

has been explored extensively as a strategy for the treatment of a variety of cancers.

MIF levels are elevated in many cancers, including bladder cancer, and MIF levels have been noted to increase during tumorigenesis in a mouse model of bladder cancer.[47] In addition, in a genetic knockout of MIF, BBN mice with NMIBC were noted to have smaller tumors with decreased tumor-associated angiogenesis and stage arrest. Furthermore, in the mouse model of NMIBC, the use of the small-molecule inhibitor CPSI-1306 reduced phosphorylated extracellular receptor kinase levels, cellular proliferation, and expression of vascular endothelial growth factor in vitro.[48]

In the same BBN carcinogen mouse model noted previously, CPSI-1306 resulted in approximately 60% reduction in tumor volume, stage migration to lower stages, and a significant reduction in proliferative indices with a trend toward decreased angiogenesis.[48] These findings were confirmed in a dose response study with no significant toxicity noted in animals. Plans for first-in-human use studies are under way pending pharmacokinetic/dynamic optimization of the inhibitor.

SUMMARY

Patients with high-grade NMIBC remain one of the most challenging group of patients for urologists to treat. High-risk patients such as those who fail to respond or recur after BCG are especially problematic. Although RC remains the standard of care for patients who fail BCG, many patients have comorbidities that make them poor candidates for cystectomy. Therefore, there remains an unmet need for effective therapies in this group. Further studies into the mechanism of resistance to BCG may provide avenues that may advance our understanding of this climate, allowing for precision medicine and targeted patient selection; however, currently, there is no evidence-based management algorithm for salvage intravesical therapy in patients with NMIBC who fail BCG therapy. The literature described previously offers promising salvage treatment regimens, but the variable methodology makes a direct comparison difficult.

Multi-arm randomized controlled trials currently under way to directly compare these treatment modalities are crucial to define optimal therapies. Current studies are limited secondary to retrospective nature, small cohort sizes, and heterogeneous cohorts of variable risk categories. There are multiple salvage options being used that add an additional layer of complexity given the varying patient populations studied with each treatment regimen with respect to age, grade, stage, number of prior BCG failures, and time to recurrence.

The good news is that there is currently a great deal of investigation and interest in identification of novel targets for therapies aimed at treating NMIBC. Recent panels with the FDA have attempted to outline the proper patient populations for testing as well as defining response. Early studies in bench to bedside therapies show promise and have the potential to provide additional options in the armamentarium against bladder cancer.

The decision to proceed with salvage intravesical therapy for NMIBC or which one, in what combination, as opposed to radical surgery with cystectomy, remains a difficult discussion for patients and urologists because of the variability in patient preference, limited high-level evidence, and an increasing number of bladder-sparing therapies. Future randomized clinical trials are necessary to determine the optimal treatment regimens for NMIBC. Interim results are encouraging and select approaches might be added for bladder-sparing options after BCG failure in the future.

REFERENCES

1. Steinberg RL, Thomas LJ, O'Donnell MA, et al. Sequential intravesical gemcitabine and docetaxel for the salvage treatment of non-muscle invasive bladder cancer. Bladder Cancer 2015;1(1):65–72.
2. Herr H, Sogani P. Does early cystectomy improve the survival of patients with high risk superficial bladder tumors? J Urol 2001;166(4):1296–9.
3. Chang SS, Boorjian SA, Chou R, et al. Diagnosis and treatment of non-muscle invasive bladder cancer: AUA/SUO guideline 2016. J Urol 2016;196(4):1021–9.
4. Gray PJ, Fedewa SA, Shipley WU, et al. Use of potentially curative therapies for muscle-invasive bladder cancer in the United States: results from the National Cancer Data Base. Eur Urol 2013; 63(5):823–9.
5. Sylvester RJ, van der Meijden AP, Witjes JA, et al. Bacillus Calmette-Guerin versus chemotherapy for the intravesical treatment of patients with carcinoma in situ of the bladder: a meta-analysis of the published results of randomized clinical trials. J Urol 2005;174(1):86–91 [discussion: 91–2].
6. Bui T, Schellhammer P. Additional bacillus Calmette-Guérin therapy for recurrent transitional cell carcinoma after an initial complete response. Urology 1997;49(5):687–91.
7. Catalona WJ, Hudson MA, Gillen DP, et al. Risks and benefits of repeated courses of intravesical bacillus Calmette-Guerin therapy for superficial bladder cancer. J Urol 1987;137(2):220–4.
8. Malmström PU, Wijkström H, Lundholm C, et al. 5-year followup of a randomized prospective study comparing mitomycin C and bacillus Calmette-Guerin in patients with superficial bladder carcinoma. Swedish-Norwegian Bladder Cancer Study Group. J Urol 1999;161(4):1124–7.
9. Steinberg G, Bahnson R, Brosman S, et al. Efficacy and safety of valrubicin for the treatment of Bacillus Calmette-Guerin refractory carcinoma in situ of the bladder. The Valrubicin Study Group. J Urol 2000; 163(3):761–7.
10. Lerner SP, Dinney C, Kamat A, et al. Clarification of bladder cancer disease states following treatment of patients with intravesical BCG. Bladder Cancer 2015;1(1):29–30.
11. Cookson MS, Chang SS, Lihou C, et al. Use of intravesical valrubicin in clinical practice for treatment of nonmuscle-invasive bladder cancer, including carcinoma in situ of the bladder. Ther Adv Urol 2014;6(5):181–91.
12. Dalbagni G, Russo P, Bochner B, et al. Phase II trial of intravesical gemcitabine in bacille Calmette-Guerin-refractory transitional cell carcinoma of the bladder. J Clin Oncol 2006;24(18):2729–34.
13. Skinner EC, Goldman B, Sakr WA, et al. SWOG S0353: phase II trial of intravesical gemcitabine in patients with nonmuscle invasive bladder cancer and recurrence after 2 prior courses of intravesical bacillus Calmette-Guerin. J Urol 2013;190(4):1200–4.

14. Di Lorenzo G, Perdonà S, Damiano R, et al. Gemcitabine versus bacille Calmette-Guerin after initial bacille Calmette-Guerin failure in non-muscle-invasive bladder cancer: a multicenter prospective randomized trial. Cancer 2010;116(8):1893–900.

15. Addeo R, Caraglia M, Bellini S, et al. Randomized phase III trial on gemcitabine versus mytomicin in recurrent superficial bladder cancer: evaluation of efficacy and tolerance. J Clin Oncol 2010;28(4): 543–8.

16. Barlow LJ, McKiernan JM, Benson MC. Long-term survival outcomes with intravesical docetaxel for recurrent nonmuscle invasive bladder cancer after previous bacillus Calmette-Guerin therapy. J Urol 2013;189(3):834–9.

17. McKiernan JM, Holder DD, Ghandour RA, et al. Phase II trial of intravesical nanoparticle albumin bound paclitaxel for the treatment of nonmuscle invasive urothelial carcinoma of the bladder after bacillus Calmette-Guerin treatment failure. J Urol 2014; 192(6):1633–8.

18. Cockerill PA, Knoedler JJ, Frank I, et al. Intravesical gemcitabine in combination with mitomycin C as salvage treatment in recurrent non-muscle-invasive bladder cancer. BJU Int 2016;117(3):456–62.

19. Lightfoot AJ, Breyer BN, Rosevear HM, et al. Multi-institutional analysis of sequential intravesical gemcitabine and mitomycin C chemotherapy for non-muscle invasive bladder cancer. Urol Oncol 2014; 32(1):35.e15-9.

20. Ryan AA, Wozniak TM, Shklovskaya E, et al. Improved protection against disseminated tuberculosis by Mycobacterium bovis bacillus Calmette-Guerin secreting murine GM-CSF is associated with expansion and activation of APCs. J Immunol 2007;179(12):8418–24.

21. Steinberg RL, Nepple KG, Velaer KN, et al. Quadruple immunotherapy of Bacillus Calmette-Guerin, interferon, interleukin-2, and granulocyte-macrophage colony-stimulating factor as salvage therapy for non-muscle-invasive bladder cancer. Urol Oncol 2017;35(12):670.e7-14.

22. Weiss C, Wolze C, Engehausen DG, et al. Radiochemotherapy after transurethral resection for high-risk T1 bladder cancer: an alternative to intravesical therapy or early cystectomy? J Clin Oncol 2006;24(15):2318–24.

23. Wo JY, Shipley WU, Dahl DM, et al. The results of concurrent chemo-radiotherapy for recurrence after treatment with bacillus Calmette-Guerin for non-muscle-invasive bladder cancer: is immediate cystectomy always necessary? BJU Int 2009;104(2): 179–83.

24. Fung CY, Shipley WU, Young RH, et al. Prognostic factors in invasive bladder carcinoma in a prospective trial of preoperative adjuvant chemotherapy and radiotherapy. J Clin Oncol 1991;9(9):1533–42.

25. Lerner SP, Bajorin DF, Dinney CP, et al. Summary and recommendations from the National Cancer Institute's clinical trials planning meeting on novel therapeutics for non-muscle invasive bladder cancer. Bladder Cancer 2016;2(2):165–202.

26. Liem EI, Crezee H, de la Rosette JJ, et al. Chemohyperthermia in non-muscle-invasive bladder cancer: an overview of the literature and recommendations. Int J Hyperthermia 2016;32(4):363–73.

27. Rampersaud E. Hyperthermia as treatment for bladder cancer. Oncology 2010;24(12):1149–55.

28. Babjuk M, Burger M, Compérat EM, et al. European Association of Urology Guidelines on Non-muscle-invasive Bladder Cancer (TaT1 and Carcinoma In Situ) - 2019 Update. Eur Urol 2019;76(5):639–57.

29. Zargar H, Aning J, Ischia J, et al. Optimizing intravesical mitomycin C therapy in non-muscle-invasive bladder cancer. Nat Rev Urol 2014;11(4): 220–30.

30. Kiss B, Schneider S, Thalmann GN, et al. Is thermochemotherapy with the Synergo system a viable treatment option in patients with recurrent non-muscle-invasive bladder cancer? Int J Urol 2015; 22(2):158–62.

31. Colombo R, Salonia A, Leib Z, et al. Long-term outcomes of a randomized controlled trial comparing thermochemotherapy with mitomycin-C alone as adjuvant treatment for non-muscle-invasive bladder cancer (NMIBC). BJU Int 2011;107(6):912–8.

32. Nativ O, Witjes JA, Hendricksen K, et al. Combined thermo-chemotherapy for recurrent bladder cancer after bacillus Calmette-Guerin. J Urol 2009;182(4): 1313–7.

33. van der Heijden AG, Kiemeney LA, Gofrit ON, et al. Preliminary European results of local microwave hyperthermia and chemotherapy treatment in intermediate or high risk superficial transitional cell carcinoma of the bladder. Eur Urol 2004;46(1): 65–71 [discussion: 71–2].

34. Alfred Witjes J, Hendricksen K, Gofrit O, et al. Intravesical hyperthermia and mitomycin-C for carcinoma in situ of the urinary bladder: experience of the European Synergo working party. World J Urol 2009;27(3):319–24.

35. Kamat AM, Colombel M, Sundi D, et al. BCG-unresponsive non-muscle-invasive bladder cancer: recommendations from the IBCG. Nat Rev Urol 2017; 14(4):244–55.

36. Racioppi M, Di Gianfrancesco L, Ragonese M, et al. ElectroMotive drug administration (EMDA) of Mitomycin C as first-line salvage therapy in high risk "BCG failure" non muscle invasive bladder cancer: 3 years follow-up outcomes. BMC Cancer 2018; 18(1):1224.

37. Burke JM, Lamm DL, Meng MV, et al. A first in human phase 1 study of CG0070, a GM-CSF expressing oncolytic adenovirus, for the treatment of

nonmuscle invasive bladder cancer. J Urol 2012; 188(6):2391–7.

38. Packiam VT, Lamm DL, Barocas DA, et al. An open label, single-arm, phase II multicenter study of the safety and efficacy of CG0070 oncolytic vector regimen in patients with BCG-unresponsive non-muscle-invasive bladder cancer: interim results. Urol Oncol 2018; 36(10):440–7.

39. Dinney CP, Fisher MB, Navai N, et al. Phase I trial of intravesical recombinant adenovirus mediated interferon-alpha2b formulated in Syn3 for Bacillus Calmette-Guerin failures in nonmuscle invasive bladder cancer. J Urol 2013;190(3):850–6.

40. Shore ND, Boorjian SA, Canter DJ, et al. Intravesical rAd-IFNα/Syn3 for patients with high-grade, bacillus Calmette-Guerin-refractory or relapsed non-muscle-invasive bladder cancer: a phase II randomized study. J Clin Oncol 2017;35(30):3410–6.

41. Hassler MR, Shariat SF, Soria F. Salvage therapeutic strategies for bacillus Calmette-Guerin failure. Curr Opin Urol 2019;29(3):239–46.

42. Kowalski M, Entwistle J, Cizeau J, et al. A Phase I study of an intravesically administered immunotoxin targeting EpCAM for the treatment of nonmuscle-invasive bladder cancer in BCGrefractory and BCG-intolerant patients. Drug Des Devel Ther 2010;4:313–20.

43. Weir SJ, Wood R, Ham T, et al. Preclinical development of ciclopirox prodrug for the treatment of non-muscle invasive and muscle invasive bladder cancer. J Clin Oncol 2018;36(15_suppl):e14576.

44. Weir SJ, Wood R, Baltezor MJ, et al. Pharmacokinetics of ciclopirox prodrug, a novel agent for the treatment of bladder cancer, in animals and humans. J Clin Oncol 2019;37(15_suppl):e14705.

45. Weir SL, Wood R, Ham T, et al. Safety, dose tolerance, pharmacokinetics and pharmacodynamics study of CPX-POM in patients with advanced solid tumors. J Clin Oncol 2018;36(15_suppl):TPS2618.

46. Penticuff J, Woolbright BL, Sielecki T, et al. Macrophage migration inhibitory factors role in genitourinary malignancies and potential for therapeutic targeting. Nat Rev Urol 2019 May;16(5):318–28.

47. Taylor JA, Voznesensky O, Kuchel GA, et al. Null mutation for macrophage migration inhibitory factor (MIF) is associated with less aggressive bladder cancer in mice. BMC Cancer 2006;7:135.

48. Choudhary S, Hegde P, Pruitt JR, et al. Macrophage Migratory Inhibitory Factor (MIF) promotes bladder cancer progression via increasing proliferation and angiogenesis. Carcinogenesis 2013;34(12):2891–9.

Moving?

Make sure your subscription moves with you!

To notify us of your new address, find your **Clinics Account Number** (located on your mailing label above your name), and contact customer service at:

Email: journalscustomerservice-usa@elsevier.com

800-654-2452 (subscribers in the U.S. & Canada)
314-447-8871 (subscribers outside of the U.S. & Canada)

Fax number: 314-447-8029

Elsevier Health Sciences Division
Subscription Customer Service
3251 Riverport Lane
Maryland Heights, MO 63043

*To ensure uninterrupted delivery of your subscription,
please notify us at least 4 weeks in advance of move.

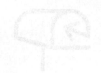

Printed and bound in CPI Group (UK) Ltd, Croydon, CR0 4YY

Printed and bound by CPI Group (UK) Ltd, Croydon, CR0 4YY

03/10/2024

01040308-0015